THE ULTIMATE GUIDE TO BUDGET-FRIENDLY PLANT-BASED MEALS: DELICIOUS, EASY, AND AFFORDABLE RECIPES FOR EVERY DAY LIFE.

BY MARYANN D. LANG

COPYRIGHT

DISCLAIMER

The information contained in this book is for general informational purposes only. While every effort has been made to ensure that the content is accurate and up-to-date, the author makes no representations or warranties of any kind, express or implied, about the completeness, accuracy, reliability, suitability, or availability with respect to the information, products, services, or related graphics contained in this book for any purpose.

Any reliance you place on such information is therefore strictly at your own risk. In no event will the author be liable for any loss or damage including without limitation, indirect or consequential loss or damage, or any loss or damage whatsoever arising from loss of data or profits arising out of, or in connection with, the use of this book.

Every effort is made to keep the book up and running smoothly. However, the author takes no responsibility for, and will not be liable for, the book being temporarily unavailable due to technical issues beyond our control.

ABOUT THE AUTHOR

Maryann D. Lang, a passionate advocate for plant-based living, presents "The Ultimate Guide to Budget-Friendly Plant-Based Meals: Delicious, Easy, and Affordable Recipes for Everyday Life." In this comprehensive cookbook, Lang offers a diverse collection of mouthwatering recipes designed to make plant-based eating accessible to everyone. From hearty main dishes to satisfying snacks and desserts, Lang's book provides delicious and nutritious options that won't break the bank. Whether you're a seasoned vegan or just starting to explore plant-based eating, this guide is sure to inspire you to create flavorful meals that are both wallet-friendly and good for you.

TABLE OF CONTENTS

Protein is an essential building block for our bodies, having a vital role in everything from muscle building and repair to hormone regulation and cell function. While many link protein with animal sources, the

Remember, this is just a starting point! With a little creativity, you can discover endless ways to add

INTRODUCTION: DELICIOUSLY AFFORDABLE PLANT-BASED EATING FOR EVERYONE

Don't forget the time you went food shopping and wished your wallet would hug you? Yes, I agree. At first, it looked like eating healthy would cost a lot. And let's be honest, who wants to spend a lot of money just to make a good meal? That's where my journey with plant-based cooking on a budget started.

It wasn't always bright and sunny. At first, all the complicated recipes and pricey items made me feel overwhelmed. Then something became clear. Without taking out a second mortgage, I found a treasure trove of tasty and healthy meals. It turns out, plant-based eating can be incredibly cheap, and trust me, it doesn't have to be bland or boring!

This book is for people who want to:

You can eat better without spending a lot of money: We'll explore clever shopping strategies, budget-friendly staples, and creative ways to stretch your food dollars further.

Fuel your body with delicious plant-based meals: We'll ditch the complicated recipes and focus on easy-to-make, flavor-packed dishes that are great for busy weeknights.

Discover the fun of plant-based cooking: Forget feeling restricted! We'll discover a world of culinary possibilities that are good for you and good for your wallet.

This guide is packed with practical tips, budget-conscious recipes, and food prep strategies that will empower you to take charge of your health and your finances. So, whether you're a seasoned cook or just starting out, join me on this delicious journey! Let's ditch the sticker shock and unlock a world of colorful, affordable plant-based meals that will leave you feeling satisfied and empowered.

Are you ready to change your kitchen and your health? Let's get started!

PART 1: POWER UP ON A BUDGET - HIGH-PROTEIN PLANT-BASED MEALS

Plant-based eating is great for your health, but sometimes the worry about getting enough protein can hold you back. Luckily, the plant world is filled with protein powerhouses, and tofu takes center stage in this chapter!

Tofu, a versatile and budget-friendly ingredient made from soybeans, is a complete protein, meaning it includes all nine important amino acids your body needs. It's also incredibly flexible, soaking up the flavors of whatever you cook it with.

This chapter will show you how to turn tofu into a wonderful and satisfying breakfast scramble packed with protein and flavor. We'll explore three versions – a classic scramble, a spicy fiesta version, and a creamy curried coconut scramble – to kickstart your day the plant-based way!

Tofu Takes Center Stage: Practical Tips

Before we dig into the recipes, let's explore some helpful tips for getting the most out of your tofu:

1. Choosing Your Tofu: Tofu comes in different forms – silken, soft, firm, and extra-firm. For scrambles, firm or extra-firm tofu works best. It holds its shape better and gives a more "eggy" texture when broken.
2. Pressing Out the Moisture: Tofu can hold a lot of water, which can

make your scramble mushy. To avoid this, press the tofu. There are fancy tofu presses available, but you can easily achieve the same effects at home. Wrap the tofu block in a clean kitchen towel or paper towel, place it on a cutting board, and weigh it down with a heavy object (like a pot or a stack of cookbooks) for about 15-20 minutes.

3. Crumbling the Tofu: Once pressed, crumble the tofu with your hands or a fork. You can aim for a coarse or finer crumble based on your preference. A finer crumble will mimic mixed eggs more closely.

4. Marinating (Optional): Marinating gives extra flavor to your tofu. Simply cube or crumble the tofu

and throw it in a bowl with your favorite marinade for at least 15 minutes. You can use a simple marinade of soy sauce, garlic powder, and ginger, or get creative with ingredients like lime juice, chipotle peppers in adobo sauce, or your favorite curry paste.

Classic Tofu Scramble (Serves 2):

This basic scramble is a great starting point and can be easily customized with your favorite add-ins.

Ingredients:

1 block (14 oz) firm or extra-firm tofu, pressed and broken

1 tablespoon olive oil

1/2 cup chopped onion

1/2 cup chopped bell pepper (any color)

1/4 cup chopped mushrooms (optional)

1/4 teaspoon turmeric powder

1/4 teaspoon smoked pepper

1/4 teaspoon garlic powder

Salt and black pepper to taste

1/4 cup chopped fresh parsley (optional)

2 tablespoons healthy yeast (optional)

Instructions:

1. Heat olive oil in a large skillet over average heat. Add the onion, bell pepper, and mushrooms (if using) and cook until softened, about 5 minutes.

2. Add the broken tofu and spices (turmeric, paprika, garlic powder) to the pan. Cook for another 5 minutes, stirring occasionally, to allow the tofu to brown slightly and absorb the flavors.

3. Season with salt and pepper to taste.

4. (Optional) Stir in the chopped fresh parsley and nutritional yeast for added flavor and nutrients.

5. Serve quickly with your favorite breakfast sides, like toast, avocado slices, or roasted vegetables.

Spicy Fiesta Tofu Scramble (Serves 2):

This version adds a kick of spice to your morning routine!

Ingredients:

1 block (14 oz) firm or extra-firm tofu, pressed and broken

1 tablespoon olive oil

1/2 cup chopped onion

1/2 cup chopped green bell pepper

1/4 cup chopped jalapeno pepper (seeds and skin removed for less heat)

1/4 cup chopped fresh cilantro

1 teaspoon chili spice

1/2 teaspoon smoked pepper

1/4 teaspoon cumin

Salt and black pepper to taste

1/4 cup crumbled vegan cheese (optional)

1 tablespoon chopped fresh lime juice (optional)

Instructions:

Follow steps 1-3 from the Classic Tofu Scramble recipe.

1. Stir in the chopped fresh cilantro and season with salt and pepper to taste.
2. (Optional) Top with crumbled vegan cheese and a squeeze of fresh lime juice for extra taste and creaminess.
3. Serve quickly with your favorite breakfast

CHAPTER 2: LENTIL LOVE: HEARTY, HEALTHY, AND BUDGET-FRIENDLY MEALS

Lentils are tiny nutritional powerhouses that deserve a starring part in your plant-based kitchen. Packed with protein, fiber, iron, and other essential nutrients, they're a budget-friendly way to make hearty and satisfying meals. Plus, lentils are highly versatile and can be enjoyed in soups, stews, salads, and even burgers!

This chapter praises lentil love with three delicious recipes:

1. **Hearty Lentil Soup with Vegetables:** A classic comfort food that's great for chilly nights.

2. **French Lentil Stew with Herbs:** A lighter and flavorful choice packed with fresh herbs.

3. **Spiced Lentil Dal with Coconut Milk:** A warm and cozy Indian-inspired dish.

Let's discover the wonderful world of lentils and unlock the potential for delicious and affordable meals!

Lentil Love: Practical Tips

Before going into the recipes, here are some helpful tips for getting the most out of your lentils:

Choosing Your Lentils: There are several types of lentils available, each with slightly different textures and cooking times. Brown lentils are the most popular type and work well in most recipes. Green lentils hold their shape well after cooking, making them great for salads or stews. Red lentils cook the fastest and break down easily, making a thicker soup texture.

Rinsing vs. Soaking: While rinsing lentils is generally recommended to remove any debris, soaking isn't always required. Brown and green lentils benefit from a 30-minute soak to shorten their cooking time. Red lentils don't require soaking and cook very quickly.

Spicing Up Your Lentils: Lentils are a blank canvas for taste! Experiment with different herbs and spices to make a variety of taste profiles. Popular choices include cumin, cilantro, turmeric, paprika, and chili powder.

Leftover Magic: Lentil recipes often taste even better the next day, as the flavors meld together. Cooked lentils can be saved in an airtight container in the refrigerator for up to 5 days. They're great for meal prep or quick lunches throughout the week.

Hearty Lentil Soup with Vegetables (Serves 4-6):

This classic soup is a crowd-pleasing choice that's perfect for a satisfying and budget-friendly meal.

Ingredients:

•1 cup brown beans, rinsed

•4 cups vegetarian broth 1 tablespoon olive oil

•1 medium onion, chopped 2 cloves garlic, minced

•2 carrots, chopped 2 celery stalks, chopped

•1 cup chopped tomatoes (fresh or canned)

•1 teaspoon dried thyme

•1/2 teaspoon dried rosemary

•1 bay leaf

•Salt and black pepper to taste

•1 cup chopped kale or spinach (optional)

•Chopped fresh parsley (optional) for garnish

Instructions:

1•In a major pot, heat olive oil over medium intensity. Add the onion and cook until relaxed, around 5 minutes.

2•Add the garlic, carrots, and celery and cook for an additional 2-3 minutes, until slightly softened.

Stir in the rinsed lentils, veggie broth, tomatoes, thyme, rosemary, and bay leaf. Bring to a boil, then reduce heat and simmer for 25-30 minutes, or until the lentils are soft.

4•(Optional) In the last few minutes of cooking, add the kale or spinach and cook until wilting.

5•Season with salt and pepper to taste.

6•Remove the bay leaf before serving.

7•Garnish with chopped fresh parsley (optional) and enjoy hot with toasted bread.

French Lentil Stew with Herbs (Serves 4-6):

This lighter and flavorful stew is packed with fresh herbs and great for a spring or summer meal.

Ingredients:

•1 cup green beans, rinsed

•4 cups vegetarian broth 1 tablespoon olive oil

•1 medium onion, chopped 2 cloves garlic, minced

•1 cup chopped zucchini

•1 cup chopped yellow squash

•1 (14.5 oz) can diced tomatoes, undrained

•1 tablespoon chopped fresh thyme

•1 tablespoon chopped fresh parsley

•1 teaspoon dried oregano

•Salt and black pepper to taste

•1/4 cup crumbled feta cheese (optional)

Instructions:

1•In a major pot, heat olive oil over medium intensity. Add the onion and cook until relaxed, around 5 minutes.

2•Add the garlic, zucchini, and yellow squash and cook for an additional 2-3 minutes, until slightly softened.

3•Stir in the rinsed lentils, veggie broth, diced tomatoes (undrained), thyme, parsley, oregano, and a pinch of salt. Bring to a boil, then reduce heat and simmer for 20-25 minutes, or until the lentils are soft but still hold their shape.

4. Season with extra salt and pepper to taste.

5. (Optional) Top individual bowls with chopped feta cheese before serving.

Spiced Lentil Dal with Coconut Milk (Serves 4-6):

This warm and comforting Indian-inspired dish is bursting with flavor and great for a cozy night in.

Ingredients:

•1 cup red lentils, washed

•4 cups vegetable broth

•1 tablespoon olive oil

•1 medium onion, chopped

•2 cloves garlic, minced

•1 teaspoon crushed cumin

•1 teaspoon chopped coriander

•1/2 teaspoon turmeric

•1 (14.5 oz) can diced tomatoes, undrained

•1 (13.5 oz) can coconut milk (light or full-fat)

•1 tablespoon chopped fresh cilantro

•1 teaspoon lime juice

•Salt and black pepper to taste

•Cooked basmati rice (optional) for serving

Instructions:

1• In a major pot, heat olive oil over medium intensity. Add the onion and cook until relaxed, around 5 minutes.

2• Add the garlic, cumin, coriander, and turmeric and cook for an additional minute, stirring constantly, to release the flavor of the spices.

3• Stir in the rinsed red lentils, veggie broth, and diced tomatoes (undrained). Bring to a boil, then reduce heat and simmer for 15-20 minutes, or until the lentils are fully softened and the mixture has thickened slightly.

4• Stir in the coconut milk, chopped cilantro, and lime juice. Season with salt and pepper to taste. Simmer for an extra 5 minutes to allow the flavors to meld.

5• Serve hot over cooked basmati rice (optional) and garnish with extra chopped fresh cilantro.

These three recipes showcase the flexibility of lentils and offer a taste of what's possible. With a little creativity, you can transform these budget-friendly legumes into delicious and satisfying meals for any event. So, embrace the lentil love and discover the endless possibilities for plant-based culinary adventures!

CHAPTER 3: BLACK BEAN BURGERS ON A BUDGET: BITE-SIZED BLISS FOR BUDGET-MINDED COOKS

Black bean burgers are a standard for a reason! They're delicious, protein-packed, and incredibly budget-friendly. Plus, they're a great way to sneak in some extra veggies for a truly well-rounded meal. This chapter dives into the world of black bean burgers, giving three variations to keep your taste buds happy:

1• **The Ultimate Black Bean Burger:** A classic and satisfying recipe that's easy to adjust.

2• **Spicy Black Bean and Quinoa** Burgers: For those who like a little heat, this version adds a kick of spice.

3• **Black Bean and Corn Burgers with Avocado Crema:** A fresh and flavorful choice with a creamy avocado topping.

Get ready to ditch the store-bought patties and make delicious black bean burgers from scratch – your wallet and your taste buds will thank you!

Black Bean Burgers on a Budget: Practical Tips

Before we dig into the recipes, let's explore some helpful tips for crafting the perfect black bean burger:

1• **Choosing Your Beans:** Canned black beans are the most convenient choice. Look for low-sodium versions to control your sodium intake.

2• **Draining and Rinsing:** Rinsing the beans helps remove excess starch and stops the burgers from becoming mushy. Drain and rinse the beans thoroughly before using them.

3• **Mashing vs. Processing:** You can either mash the beans with a fork for a chunkier texture or use a food processor for a softer consistency. It's a matter of personal taste!

4• **Binding Power:** Eggs are a popular binder in burgers, but there are vegan-friendly alternatives. Mashed flaxseed meal mixed with water, mashed sweet potato or cooking quinoa can all act as binders.

5• **Flavor Boosters:** Don't be shy with the spices! Cumin, chili powder, smoked paprika, garlic powder, and onion powder are all excellent choices to add depth of flavor to your burgers.

6• Forming the Patties: Use your hands to gently form the burger mixture into patties. Aim for a thickness of about 3/4 inch to 1 inch to keep them from falling apart during cooking.

7• Cooking Methods: You can cook your black bean burgers in a pan on the stovetop, grill them outdoors, or even bake them in the oven. Each method offers slightly different textures – try to find your favorite!

The Ultimate Black Bean Burger (Serves 4):

This standard recipe is a great starting point for your black bean burger adventures. Feel free to get artistic and customize it with your favorite add-ins!

Ingredients:

•1 (15 oz) can black beans, drained and washed

•1/2 cup cooked brown rice

•1/4 cup chopped red onion

•1/4 cup chopped fresh cilantro

•1 tablespoon olive oil

•1 tablespoon lemon juice

•1 tablespoon ground cumin

•1/2 teaspoon chili spice

•1/2 teaspoon smoked pepper

•1/4 teaspoon garlic powder

•1/4 teaspoon onion powder

•1/4 cup panko breadcrumbs (or rolled oats)

•Salt and black pepper to taste

•Hamburger buns (extra)

•Toppings of your choice (e.g., lettuce, tomato, sliced avocado, vegan cheese)

Instructions:

1• In a large bowl, mash the black beans with a fork or pulse them a few times in a food processor until a slightly chunky mixture is achieved. You don't want them completely smooth.

2• Add the cooked brown rice, chopped onion, chopped cilantro, olive oil, lemon juice, spices (cumin, chili powder, paprika, garlic powder, onion powder), and breadcrumbs to the mashed beans.

3• Season with salt and pepper to taste. Mix well to mix all ingredients.

4• Form the mixture into 4 equal-sized patties, about 3/4 inch to 1 inch thick.

5• Heat a pan over medium heat with a drizzle of olive oil.

6• Cook the burger patties for 3-4 minutes per side, or until golden brown and warm through.

7• Serve on hamburger buns (optional) with your favorite toppings like lettuce, tomato, sliced avocado, vegan cheese, or your best burger sauce.

Spicy Black Bean and Quinoa Burgers (Serves 4):

Like a little heat? This version adds a kick of spice to your black bean burger game!

Ingredients:

•1 (15 oz) can black beans, drained and washed

•1/2 cup cooked quinoa

•1/4 cup chopped red onion

•1/4 cup chopped jalapeno pepper (seeds and skin removed for less heat)

•1 tablespoon olive oil

•1 tablespoon lime juice

•1 tablespoon chopped fresh cilantro

•1 teaspoon crushed cumin

•1/2 teaspoon chili spice

•1/2 teaspoon smoked pepper

•1/4 teaspoon garlic powder

•1/4 teaspoon onion powder

•1/4 teaspoon cayenne pepper (adjust to your spice taste)

•1/4 cup rolled oats

•Salt and black pepper to taste

•Hamburger buns (extra)

•Toppings of your choice (e.g., lettuce, tomato, sliced avocado, vegan cheese, vegan cream)

Instructions:

1• Follow steps 1-4 from The Ultimate Black Bean Burger recipe, using the listed items for this spicy version.

2• Be sure to include the chopped jalapeno pepper for that spicy kick. Adjust the amount according to your chosen heat level.

3• Form the mixture into 4 equal-sized patties, about 3/4 inch to 1 inch thick.

4• Heat a pan over medium heat with a drizzle of olive oil.

5• Cook the burger patties for 3-4 minutes per side, or until golden brown and warm through.

6• Serve on hamburger buns (optional) with your favorite toppings like lettuce, tomato, sliced avocado, vegan cheese, or vegan cream.

Black Bean and Corn Burgers with Avocado Crema (Serves 4):

This version offers a fresh and flavorful change with the addition of corn and a creamy avocado topping.

Ingredients:

•1 (15 oz) can black beans, drained and washed

•1/2 cup cooked brown rice

•1/2 cup frozen corn, thawed and drained

- 1/4 cup chopped red onion
- 1/4 cup chopped fresh cilantro
- 1 tablespoon olive oil
- 1 tablespoon lime juice
- 1 tablespoon ground cumin
- 1/2 teaspoon chili spice
- 1/2 teaspoon smoked pepper
- 1/4 teaspoon garlic powder
- 1/4 teaspoon onion powder
- 1/4 cup panko breadcrumbs (or rolled oats)
- Salt and black pepper to taste
- Hamburger buns (extra)
- Toppings of your choice (e.g., lettuce, tomato)

For the Avocado Crema:

- 1 ripe avocado, mashed
- 1/4 cup chopped fresh cilantro
- 1 tablespoon lime juice
- Salt and black pepper to taste

Instructions:

1• In a large bowl, mash the black beans with a fork or pulse them a few times in a food processor until a slightly chunky mixture is achieved.

2• Add the cooked brown rice, thawed and drained corn, chopped onion, chopped cilantro, olive oil, lime juice, spices (cumin, chili powder, paprika, garlic powder, onion powder), and breadcrumbs to the mashed beans.

3• Season with salt and pepper to taste. Mix well to mix all ingredients.

4• Form the mixture into 4 equal-sized patties, about 3/4 inch to 1 inch thick.

5• Heat a pan over medium heat with a drizzle of olive oil.

6• Cook the burger patties for 3-4 minutes per side, or until golden brown and warm through.

For the Avocado Crema:

In a small bowl, mix the mashed avocado, chopped cilantro, lime juice, salt, and pepper. Mash until smooth and creamy.

To Assemble:

1• Serve the black bean and corn burgers on hamburger buns (optional) with your favorite additions like lettuce and tomato.

2• Top each burger with a dollop of the creamy avocado crema.

These three black bean burger variations showcase the versatility and deliciousness of this budget-friendly choice. So, fire up the grill, preheat the oven, or heat up your skillet, and get ready to experience the joy of making and enjoying homemade black bean burgers!

CHAPTER 4: PLANT-BASED PROTEIN POWERHOUSE: A GUIDE TO POWERING UP YOUR MEALS

Protein is an essential building block for our bodies, having a vital role in everything from muscle building and repair to hormone regulation and cell function. While many link protein with animal sources, the plant-based world offers a treasure trove of protein-rich options to keep you fueled and feeling your best.

This chapter dives into a range of plant-based protein powerhouses, exploring their versatility and nutritional benefits:

•The Many Uses of Beans and Lentils:

We already covered these powerhouses in Chapter 2, but here's a deeper look at their versatility.

•Tempeh: A Versatile Protein Option:

This fermented soybean cake is packed with protein and great for adding variety to your meals.

•Exploring Other Plant-Based Protein Sources:

We'll venture beyond the usual suspects to find additional protein-rich options from the plant kingdom.

Get ready to unlock the full potential of plant-based protein and make delicious and satisfying meals that nourish your body!

Plant-Based Protein Powerhouse: Practical Tips

Before we dig into specific protein sources, here are some helpful tips for incorporating more plant-based protein into your diet:

•Variety is Key: Don't depend on just one or two protein sources. Mix and match throughout the week to ensure you're getting a full range of amino acids.

•Combine Protein with Grains: Pairing protein sources with whole grains like brown rice, quinoa, or whole-wheat bread creates a complete protein, meaning it includes all nine essential amino acids your body needs.

•Planning Makes Perfect: Planning your meals and snacks in advance can help ensure you're getting enough protein throughout the day.

•**Don't Forget the Greens:** Leafy green vegetables like spinach and kale also contain some protein, and they're loaded with other important nutrients.

The Many Uses of Beans and Lentils:

As you already know from Chapter 2, beans and lentils are protein powerhouses that are budget-friendly and incredibly flexible. Let's explore some ways to combine these staples into your diet beyond hearty soups and stews:

•**Salads:** Add cooked and cooled beans or lentils to salads for a protein boost and extra crunch.

•**Burgers:** We studied black bean burgers in Chapter 3, but don't stop there! Experiment with other beans and lentils in your burger recipes.

•**Pasta Sauce:** Bulk up your pasta sauce by adding cooked and mashed beans or lentils.

•**Dips and Spreads:** Mashed beans or lentils can be turned into delicious and protein-rich dips and spreads for crackers or crudités.

Tempeh: A Versatile Protein Option:

Tempeh is a fermented soybean cake with a slightly nutty taste and a firm texture. It's a great source of protein and can be marinated, crumbled, sliced, or cubed to fit your recipe needs. Here are some opinions to get you started:

•**Tempeh "Bacon":** Marinate tempeh slices in a smoky marinade and bake or pan-fry for a delicious veggie alternative to bacon bits on salads or breakfast scrambles.

•**Tempeh Stir-Fry:** Cube tempeh and marinate it in your best sauce before stir-frying with vegetables and tofu for a protein-packed and flavorful meal.

•**Tempeh "Crumbs":** Crumble tempeh and use it as a topping for tacos, pasta recipes, or casseroles for a protein and textural boost.

Exploring Other Plant-Based Protein Sources:

Beyond beans, lentils, and tempeh, there's a whole world of plant-based protein waiting to be discovered! Here are some other protein-rich choices to consider:

•**Nuts and Seeds:** Almonds, walnuts, cashews, chia seeds, and hemp seeds are all great sources of protein and healthy fats. Enjoy them by the handful, sprinkle them on soups or yogurt, or use them to make homemade nut butters.

•**Seitan (Gluten-Free Option Available):** Made from wheat gluten, seitan has a chewy feel and can be seasoned and cooked in endless ways.
•**Important Note:** If you have celiac disease or a gluten sensitivity, avoid seitan and explore other gluten-free protein choices.

•**Nutritional Yeast:** This deactivated yeast is a nutritional powerhouse, having protein, vitamins, and minerals. Sprinkle it on popcorn, pasta dishes, or use it to add a cheesy taste to vegan mac and cheese.

•**Quinoa:** This ancient grain is a complete protein source, meaning it includes all nine essential amino acids. Use it in place of rice, or eat it in salads or breakfast bowls.

Remember, this is just a starting point! With a little creativity, you can discover endless ways to add these plant-based protein sources into your meals. Don't be afraid to try and find what works best for your taste buds and dietary needs.

The Takeaway:

The plant-based world is bursting with protein powerhouses waiting to be discovered. From budget-friendly beans and lentils to the versatility of tempeh and the variety of other options, you can make delicious and satisfying meals that nourish your body and keep you feeling energized throughout the day.

Ready to take the plunge and discover the exciting world of plant-based protein? The next chapters will delve into delicious recipes featuring these protein powerhouses, giving you practical ideas to create plant-based meals that are both nutritious and mouthwatering. So, turn the page and start on a culinary adventure packed with flavor and protein!

PART 2: WEEKNIGHT WINS - QUICK AND EASY PLANT-BASED MEALS

We all know that weeknights can be crazy. With work, family, and other responsibilities, it can be hard to find the time and energy to make a tasty and healthy meal. This is where one-pot plant-based miracles come in handy!

These recipes are meant to be quick, simple, and clean up easily, making them great for busy weeknights. All of them are cooked in one pot, which cuts down on plates and speeds up the process.

CHAPTER 5 FEATURES THREE ONE-POT WONDERS THAT ARE BURSTING WITH FLAVOR:

1. Creamy Vegan Tomato Pasta (One-Pot): A comforting and filling pasta dish with a creamy tomato sauce.

2. Thai Curry Chickpea Bowl (One-Pot): A delicious and aromatic bowl packed with protein and veggies.

3. Mexican Quinoa Bake (One-Pot): A cheesy and delicious dish with a Mexican twist.

Get ready to say goodbye to takeout and hello to easy, filling plant-based meals that fit your busy schedule!

Weekday Wins: Practical Tips for One-Pot Wonders

Before we dig into the recipes, here are some helpful tips for making your one-pot wonders a success:

- **Prep is Key:** Take a few minutes to chop your veggies and gather your ingredients before starting. This will make the cooking method much easier.
- **The Power of Pantry Staples:** Stock your pantry with important items like canned beans, diced tomatoes, pasta, and rice. These ingredients can be turned into countless one-pot meals.
- **Frozen is Fantastic:** Frozen veggies are a lifesaver when it comes to quick and easy meals. They're pre-washed and chopped, saving you important time.
- **Spice Up Your Life:** Don't be afraid to try with different herbs and spices. They add taste depth and can take your one-pot wonders to the next level.
- **Leftover Love:** Many one-pot meals taste even better the next day. Cook a double batch and enjoy delicious leftovers for lunch or another quick dinner.

Creamy Vegan Tomato Pasta (One-Pot) (Serves 4):

This warm and filling pasta dish is made in a single pot, making cleanup a breeze!

Ingredients:

1 tablespoon olive oil

1 medium onion, chopped

2 cloves garlic, minced

1 (28 oz) can crushed tomatoes

1 (14.5 oz) can diced tomatoes, undrained

1 cup veggie broth

1/2 cup plain plant-based milk (e.g., almond milk, soy milk)

1 tablespoon tomato sauce

1 teaspoon dried oregano

1/2 teaspoon dried mint

1/4 teaspoon red pepper flakes (optional)

1 cup dried pasta (e.g., penne, rotini)

1 cup chopped fresh spinach or kale

Salt and black pepper to taste

Chopped fresh parsley (optional) for garnish

Instructions:

• Heat olive oil in a big pot or Dutch oven over medium heat. Put in the chopped onion and cook until it's loosened up, about 5 minutes.

• Add the minced garlic and cook for an extra minute, until fragrant.

• Stir in the crushed tomatoes, diced tomatoes (undrained), veggie broth, plant-based milk, tomato paste, oregano, basil, and red pepper flakes (if using).

• Get to a boil, then lower heat and cook for 10 minutes.

• Add the dry pasta and stir to coat with the sauce.

• Cook according to box directions for the pasta, turning occasionally, until the pasta is al dente and the sauce has thickened slightly.

• In the last few minutes of cooking, stir in the chopped spinach or kale and cook until soft.

• Season it with salt and add black pepper to taste.

• Serve immediately served with chopped fresh parsley (optional).

Thai Curry Chickpea Bowl (One-Pot) (Serves 4):

This tasty and aromatic bowl features protein-packed chickpeas in a delicious Thai curry sauce.

Ingredients:

1 tablespoon olive oil

1 halfway onion, sliced 2 cloves garlic, minced

1 tablespoon yellow curry sauce

1 (13.5 oz) can coconut milk (light or full-fat)

1 (15 oz) can chickpeas, drained and washed

1 cup vegetable broth 1 cup chopped broccoli stems

1 cup chopped red bell pepper

1/2 cup chopped green beans 1 tablespoon soy sauce

1 tablespoon lime juice

1 tablespoon chopped fresh cilantro

Cooked brown rice (optional) for serving

Lime wedges and chopped peanuts (optional) for garnish

Instructions:

• Heat olive oil in a large pot or Dutch oven over moderate heat. Put in the chopped onion and cook until softened, about 5 minutes.

• Add the minced garlic and cook for an extra minute, until fragrant.

• Stir in the yellow curry paste and cook for another minute, allowing the flavors to release.

• Pour in the coconut milk, cleaning up any browned bits from the bottom of the pot.

• Add the drained and rinsed chickpeas, veggie broth, chopped broccoli florets, red bell pepper, and green beans.

• Bring to a boil, then reduce heat and simmer for 15-20 minutes, or until the vegetables are tender-crisp and the beans are heated through.

• Stir in the soy sauce and lime juice.

• Season with salt and black pepper to taste (be aware that soy sauce can be spicy, so adjust accordingly).

• Serve hot over cooked brown rice (optional) and top with chopped fresh cilantro, lime wedges, and chopped peanuts (optional).

Mexican Quinoa Bake (One-Pot) (Serves 4):

This cheesy and delicious casserole with a Mexican twist is sure to become a family favorite!

Ingredients:

- 1 tablespoon olive oil
- 1 medium onion, chopped

- 1 green bell pepper, chopped
- 2 cloves garlic, minced
- 1 (15 oz) can black beans, rinsed and drained
- 1 (14.5 oz) can diced tomatoes, undrained
- 1 cup vegetable broth
- 1 cup uncooked quinoa, rinsed
- 1 (10 oz) can diced green chiles (mild or hot, depending on your preference)
- 1 teaspoon ground cumin
- 1/2 teaspoon chili powder
- 1/4 teaspoon smoked paprika
- 1 cup shredded vegan cheese (optional)
- Fresh cilantro, chopped avocado, and vegan sour cream (optional) for garnish

Instructions:

1. Preheat oven to 375°F (190°C).
2. Heat olive oil in a large pot or Dutch oven over medium heat. Add the chopped onion and green pepper and cook until softened, about 5 minutes.
3. Stir in the minced garlic and cook for an additional minute, until fragrant.
4. Add the rinsed and drained black beans, diced tomatoes (undrained), vegetable broth,

rinsed quinoa, diced green chiles, cumin, chili powder, and smoked paprika.

5. Bring to a boil, then reduce heat, cover, and simmer for 15 minutes, or until the quinoa is cooked through and the liquid has been absorbed.
6. Remove from heat and stir in the shredded vegan cheese (optional).
7. Transfer the mixture to a baking dish and bake for 10-15 minutes, or until the cheese is melted and bubbly (if using).
8. Serve hot garnished with chopped fresh cilantro, chopped avocado, and vegan sour cream (optional).

These three one-pot wonders demonstrate the ease and flavor potential of plant-based meals. So ditch the takeout menus, grab your favorite pot, and whip up a delicious and satisfying weeknight meal in no time!

CHAPTER 6: 30-MINUTE MEALS THAT MATTER

We all know that things can get busy. Making time to cook a healthy and tasty meal can be hard when you have a lot on your plate, like work, chores, and social plans. This chapter saves the day with a list of 30-minute meals that are full of flavor and won't keep you stuck in the kitchen.

These recipes are meant to be quick and easy, so you won't need much time to prepare or cook them. They are great for busy weeknights or any time you want a filling meal without a lot of work.

There are three tasty 30-minute meals in this chapter, each one suitable for a different taste:

Stir-Fried Vegetables with Tofu and Peanut Sauce: Tofu, veggie, and peanut sauce stir-fried in a light and tasty sauce. The vegetables are brightly colored and the tofu is high in protein.
Creamy Vegan Pasta Primavera: A pasta dish with lots of vegetables and a creamy sauce that is great for when you're wanting comfort food.

Lentil and Vegetable Curry with Roti: A fragrant and tasty curry made with protein-rich lentils that is great for a filling and unique meal.
Get ready to ditch the frozen dinners and make incredible meals in just 30 minutes!

30-Minute Meals that Matter: Practical Tips for Speed

Before we dig into the recipes, here are some helpful tips for conquering the 30-minute meal:

1. **Mise en Place:** This French term simply means "having everything in its place." Before starting, chop your veggies, measure your ingredients, and have everything prepped and ready to go. This will ease the cooking process.

2. **The Power of Pre-Chopped and Prepped:** Keep frozen chopped vegetables or pre-cut fresh options on hand to save important prep time. Look for pre-cooked choices like brown rice or quinoa to shave off additional minutes.

3. **Master the Multitasking Art:** While one thing cooks, prep another. For example, chop veggies while your rice simmers on the stove.

4. **High Heat, Short Time:** Stir-fries and other quick-cooking techniques utilize high heat for a short cooking time, keeping the vibrancy of your vegetables.

5. **Leftover Love:** Many 30-minute meals taste just as good, or even better, the next day. Cook a double batch to enjoy delicious leftovers for lunch or another quick dinner.

Stir-Fried Vegetables with Tofu and Peanut Sauce (Serves 4):

This light and flavorful stir-fry is packed with colorful veggies, protein-rich tofu, and a delicious peanut sauce.

INGREDIENTS:

1 tablespoon cornstarch
3 tablespoons soy sauce

1 tablespoon brown sugar
1 tablespoon rice vinegar
1 tablespoon sriracha (adjust to your spice taste)
1 tablespoon smooth peanut butter
1 tablespoon sesame oil
1 tablespoon olive oil
1 block firm tofu, drained and pressed (optional: cubed or broken)
1 cup assorted veggies (e.g., broccoli florets, red bell pepper strips, snow peas, carrots)
1 cup cooked brown rice (optional)
Chopped fresh parsley and peanuts (optional) for garnish

INSTRUCTIONS:

1. In a small bowl, mix together cornstarch, soy sauce, brown sugar, rice vinegar, sriracha, peanut butter, and sesame oil. Set aside.

2. Heat olive oil in a big skillet or wok over medium-high heat.

3. Add the tofu (if using) and cook until golden brown on all sides, about 5 minutes. Remove from the pan and set aside (optional).

4. Add the assorted veggies to the pan and cook, stirring frequently, for 3-4 minutes, or until crisp-tender.

5. Pour the prepared sauce mixture into the pan with the veggies and bring to a simmer.

6. If using tofu, add it back to the pan and cook for an additional minute to heat through.

7. Serve quickly over cooked brown rice (optional) and garnish with chopped fresh cilantro and peanuts (optional).

Creamy Vegan Pasta Primavera (Serves 4):

This creamy pasta dish with lots of vegetables is great for a warm and filling meal.

INGREDIENTS:

1 tablespoon olive oil

1 whole onion, cut up

Two cloves of chopped garlic

1 (14.5 oz) can diced tomatoes, not drained

1 cup veggie broth 1/2 cup unsweetened plant-based milk (e.g., almond milk, soy milk)

Half a cup of healthy yeast

1 teaspoon of cornstarch

1 teaspoon of dried oregano

1/2 teaspoon dried mint

1/4 teaspoon red pepper flakes (optional)

1 cup assorted veggies (eg., asparagus, broccoli florets, zucchini, halved cherry tomatoes)

8 ounces dried pasta (e.g., penne, rotini)

Salt and black pepper to taste

Chopped fresh parsley (optional) for garnish

INSTRUCTIONS:

1. Heat olive oil in a big pot or Dutch oven over medium heat. Add the chopped onion and cook until it loosens up, about 5 minutes.

2. Add the chopped garlic and cook for an additional minute, until fragrant.

3. Stir in the diced tomatoes (undrained), veggie broth, plant-based milk, nutritional yeast, cornstarch, oregano, basil, and red pepper flakes (if using).

4. Bring to a boil, then reduce heat and cook for 5 minutes.

5. Add the assorted veggies and cook for an additional 5-7 minutes, or until the vegetables are tender-crisp.

6. While the vegetables cook, cook the pasta according to package directions in a different pot of boiling salted water.

7. Once the pasta is cooked, drain it and add it to the pot with the sauce and veggies.

8. Season with salt and black pepper to taste.

9. Serve immediately topped with chopped fresh parsley (optional).

Lentil and Vegetable Curry with Roti (Serves 4):

This flavorful and aromatic curry features protein-packed lentils and a delicious base, perfect for a filling and exotic meal.

INGREDIENTS:

1 tablespoon olive oil
1 whole onion, cut up
Two cloves of chopped garlic
1 tablespoon curry powder
1 teaspoon crushed cumin
1/2 teaspoon turmeric
1/4 teaspoon chili sauce (optional)
1 (14.5 oz) can diced tomatoes, not drained
1 cup of veggie broth
1 cup green lentils, cleaned

1 cup chopped veggies (e.g., carrots, potatoes, green beans)
1 (10 oz) can coconut milk (light or full-fat)
Salt and black pepper to taste
Chopped fresh cilantro and store-bought roti (flatbread) for serving

INSTRUCTIONS:

1. Heat olive oil in a big pot or Dutch oven over medium heat. Add the chopped onion and cook until it loosens up, about 5 minutes.

2. Add the chopped garlic and cook for an additional minute, until fragrant.

3. Stir in the curry powder, cumin, turmeric, and chili powder (if using).
4. Cook for an additional minute, allowing the spices to release their flavor.

5. Pour in the diced tomatoes (undrained) and veggie broth.

6. Add the rinsed green lentils, chopped veggies, and coconut milk.

7. Bring to a boil, then lower heat, cover, and simmer for 20-25 minutes, or until the lentils are tender and the 8. veggies are cooked through. Season with salt and black pepper to taste.

9. Serve hot over store-bought roti flatbread and top with chopped fresh cilantro.

These 30-minute meals show the incredible potential for quick, flavorful, and satisfying plant-based dishes. With a little planning and these helpful tips, you can conquer busy weeknights without sacrificing taste or nutrition. So grab your items, set a timer, and get ready to whip up a delicious meal in no time!

CHAPTER 7: 5-INGREDIENT MAGIC: DELICIOUS MEALS IN MINUTES

Life can get busy, and sometimes the thought of cooking a healthy and satisfying meal feels overwhelming. Who has the time for complicated recipes and long ingredient lists? This chapter dives into the world of 5-ingredient magic, showing delicious and nutritious meals that can be whipped up in no time with minimal ingredients.

Here's the beauty of 5-ingredient magic:

1. Simple is Spectacular: With just a handful of ingredients, you can make restaurant-worthy dishes that are packed with flavor and good for you.

2. Pantry Staples Shine: Many of these recipes utilize ingredients you might already have on hand, lowering the need for frequent grocery trips.

3. Quick and Easy: These dishes come together in minutes, making them great for busy weeknights or when you're short on time.

Get ready to unlock the magic of simple cooking with these delicious 5-ingredient recipes:

1. Black Bean and Corn Quesadillas: A satisfying and flavorful vegetarian twist on a favorite.

2. Roasted veggies with Tahini Dressing: Simple roasted veggies transformed with a creamy and flavorful tahini dressing.

3. Creamy Tomato and Chickpea Soup: A comforting and protein-packed soup that's great for chilly nights.

4. Spicy Peanut Noodles with Tofu: This flavorful and protein-packed dish is ready in minutes, perfect for a satisfying and light meal. (New!)

5. Fruity Oatmeal Bake: A healthy and delicious twist on oatmeal, perfect for a satisfying breakfast or snack. (New!)

5-Ingredient Magic: Tips and Tricks

Before we dive into the recipes, here are some helpful tips to improve your 5-ingredient magic experience:

1. Quality Counts: While these recipes only call for a few ingredients, choose high-quality ingredients

whenever available. Fresh, flavorful fruit will elevate your dishes.

2. Seasoning is Key: Don't discount the power of salt, pepper, and other spices. They can turn simple ingredients into something truly delicious.

3. Get Creative with Toppings: While these recipes are complete on their own, feel free to add your favorite toppings for extra taste and texture. For example, add chopped avocado to your quesadillas or a dollop of vegan yogurt to your soup.

4. Leftover Love: Many 5-ingredient magic foods taste just as good, or even better, the next day. Cook a double batch to enjoy delicious leftovers for lunch or another quick dinner.

Black Bean and Corn Quesadillas (Serves 2):

These vegetarian quesadillas are packed with taste and protein, making them a quick and satisfying meal or snack.

Ingredients:

2 big whole-wheat tortillas
1 (15 oz) can black beans, drained and rinsed
1/2 cup frozen corn, thawed and drained
1/4 cup shredded cheese (optional)
Chopped fresh cilantro (optional) for garnish

Instructions:

1. Heat a big skillet or griddle over medium heat.

2. Spread half of the black beans on one tortilla. Sprinkle half of the corn and cheese (if using).

3. Fold the tortilla in half and cook for 2-3 minutes per side, or until golden brown and crispy.

4. Repeat with the leftover tortilla, black beans, corn, and cheese (if using).

5. Serve immediately topped with chopped fresh cilantro (optional).

Roasted Vegetables with Tahini Dressing (Serves 4):

Simple roasted veggies become a flavor explosion with this creamy and flavorful tahini dressing.

Ingredients:

2 tablespoons olive oil
1 pound assorted veggies (e.g., broccoli florets, red bell pepper wedges, zucchini slices)
Salt and black pepper to taste
1/4 cup tahini
2 tablespoons lemon juice
1-2 tablespoons water (optional)

Instructions:

1. Preheat the oven to 400°F (200°C).
Toss the assorted veggies with olive oil, salt, and pepper.

2. Spread the veggies on a baking sheet in a single layer.

3. Roast for 20-25 minutes, or until tender-crisp and slightly browned.

4. While the vegetables roast, make the dressing. In a small bowl, mix together tahini, lemon juice, and enough water (optional) to achieve a desired consistency (thin or thick).

5. Serve the roasted vegetables drizzled with the tahini sauce.

Creamy Tomato and Chickpea Soup (Serves 4):

This comforting and protein-packed soup is great for a quick and easy weeknight meal.

Ingredients:

1 tablespoon olive oil

1 medium onion, chopped, 2 cloves garlic, minced (28 oz) can crushed tomatoes (15 oz) can chickpeas, drained and rinsed

Salt and black pepper to taste

Instructions:

1. Heat olive oil in a big pot or Dutch oven over medium heat. Add the chopped onion and cook until it loosens up, about 5 minutes.

2. Add the chopped garlic and cook for an additional minute, until fragrant.

Pour in the blended tomatoes and bring to a simmer.

3. Add the drained and rinsed beans.

4. Spice it up with salt and black pepper to taste.

5. Reduce heat and simmer for 10–15 minutes, or until the flavors meld.

6. Using an immersion blender or moving the soup to a blender in batches, blend the soup until the desired consistency (smooth or slightly chunky).

5. Serve hot.

Spicy Peanut Noodles with Tofu (Serves 2):

This flavorful and protein-packed dish is ready in minutes, great for a satisfying and light meal.

Ingredients:

8 ounces dried noodles (e.g., rice noodles, soba noodles)

1 block firm tofu, drained and cubed

1 tablespoon soy sauce

1 tablespoon sriracha (adjust to your spice taste)

1 tablespoon smooth peanut butter

Chopped fresh peanuts and chopped fresh cilantro (optional) for garnish

Instructions:

1. Cook the noodles according to package directions.

2. While the noodles cook, heat a large pot or pan over medium heat. Add the cubed tofu and cook for 5-7 minutes per side, or until golden brown and crispy.

3. In a small bowl, mix together soy sauce, sriracha, and peanut butter.

4. Drain the cooked noodles and toss them with the prepared sauce in a big bowl.

5. Add the cooked tofu to the noodle mixture and toss to blend.

Serve immediately topped with chopped fresh peanuts and chopped fresh cilantro (optional).

Fruity Oatmeal Bake (Serves 4):

A healthy and delicious twist on oatmeal, great for a satisfying breakfast or snack.

Ingredients:

1 cup rolled oats

1 cup plain plant-based milk (e.g., almond milk, soy milk)

1 cup chopped fresh or frozen fruit (e.g., berries, mango, peaches)

1/4 cup crushed nuts or seeds (e.g., almonds, walnuts, chia seeds)

1 tablespoon maple syrup (optional)

Instructions:

1. Preheat the oven to 375°F (190°C).

In a baking dish, mix rolled oats, plant-based milk, chopped fruit, and chopped nuts or seeds.

2. Drizzle with maple syrup (optional) for extra sweetness.

3. Bake for 20-25 minutes, or until the oatmeal is set and the fruit is cooked.

Serve warm.

These 5-ingredient magic recipes show the incredible potential for quick, flavorful, and nutritious plant-based meals. With a little creativity and these handy tips, you can make delicious and satisfying dishes without spending hours in the kitchen. So stock your pantry with some basic essentials, embrace minimalist cooking, and open the world of 5-ingredient magic!

CHAPTER 8: LEFTOVER TRANSFORMATIONS: TURNING SCRAPS INTO SCRAPTASTIC MEALS

We've all been there: you cook a great meal, but there's just too much leftover. The thought of eating the same thing again tomorrow might be less than appealing. Fear not! This chapter dives into the art of leftover transformations, showing creative ways to repurpose those leftovers into exciting new dishes.

Leftover changes offer numerous benefits:

1. **Reduce Food Waste:** By using up leftovers, you're saving money and reducing food waste, which is good for your wallet and the world.
2. **Boost Creativity:** Leftovers become a springboard for culinary research. You can experiment with different flavors and ingredients to make something entirely new.
3. **Save Time and Money:** You've already cooked the main ingredient, so these recipes often come together quickly and require minimal extra shopping.

Get ready to breathe new life into your leftovers with these amazing transformation ideas:

1. **Leftover Veggie Stir-Fry with Noodles:** Give leftover roasted vegetables a tasty makeover in a quick and easy stir-fry.
2. **Lentil Soup Transformation:** Spiced Lentil Shepherd's Pie: Transform leftover lentil soup into a filling and comforting shepherd's pie.
3. **Black Bean Burger Transformation: Black Bean Burrito Bowls:** Repurpose extra black bean burgers into delicious and customizable burrito bowls.

Leftover Transformations: Tips and Tricks

Before we dive into the recipes, here are some helpful tips to improve your leftover transformation experience:

1. Storage is Key: Store leftovers properly in closed containers in the refrigerator for 3-4 days or freeze them for longer storage.

2. Think Outside the Box: Don't be afraid to get creative! Excess roasted chicken can be turned into a salad, quesadillas, or even a pot pie filling.

3. Embrace Flavor Boosters: Fresh herbs, spices, and sauces can put new life into leftovers. A squeeze of lemon juice, a sprinkle of chili flakes, or a dollop of pesto can work wonders.

4. Get Grainy: Leftover proteins and veggies pair beautifully with grains like rice, quinoa, or couscous. This makes a complete and satisfying meal.

Leftover Veggie Stir-Fry with Noodles (Serves 4):

Transform your extra roasted vegetables into a flavorful and satisfying stir-fry with this quick and easy recipe.

Ingredients:

2 tablespoons olive oil
1 clove garlic, minced
1 teaspoon chopped ginger (optional)
1-2 cups assorted leftover roasted veggies (e.g., broccoli florets, red bell pepper strips, zucchini slices)
1/2 cup chopped onion (optional, if veggies weren't cooked with onion)
1 cup cooked protein (optional, extra chicken, tofu, tempeh)
1/2 cup frozen peas (optional)
1/4 cup soy sauce

1 tablespoon brown sugar
1 tablespoon cornstarch
1 tablespoon rice vinegar
1/4 teaspoon sriracha (adjust to your spice taste)
Cooked noodles of your choice (e.g., rice noodles, soba noodles, pasta)
Chopped fresh cilantro and chopped green onions (optional) for garnish

Instructions:

1. Cook your choice of noodles according to package directions.
2. Heat olive oil in a big skillet or wok over medium-high heat. Add the chopped garlic and grated ginger (if using) and cook for 30 seconds, until fragrant.

2. Add the chopped onion (if using) and cook until softened, about 5 minutes.

3. Add the leftover roasted vegetables and cook for 2-3 minutes, stirring regularly.

4. If using cooked protein, add it to the pan and heat through.

5. In a small bowl, mix together soy sauce, brown sugar, cornstarch, rice vinegar, and sriracha.

6. Pour the sauce mixture into the pan with the veggies and protein. Bring to a boil and cook for 1-2 minutes, or until the sauce thickens slightly.

7. Serve the stir-fry over cooked noodles and top with chopped fresh cilantro and sliced green onions (optional).

Lentil Soup Transformation: Spiced Lentil Shepherd's Pie (Serves 4):

Take your leftover lentil soup to the next level with this cozy and flavorful shepherd's pie.

Ingredients:

2 tablespoons olive oil

1 medium onion, chopped

1 clove garlic, minced

1 carrot, diced (optional)

1 celery stalk, diced (optional)

1/2 cup frozen peas

1/2 teaspoon dried thyme

1/4 teaspoon dried rosemary

1/teaspoon smoked paprika (optional)

Salt and black pepper to taste

4 cups extra lentil soup

1/2 cup mashed potatoes (homemade or store-bought)

Chopped fresh parsley (optional) for garnish

Instructions:

1. Preheat the oven to 375°F (190°C).

2. Heat olive oil in a large pan or Dutch oven over medium heat. Add the chopped onion and cook until it loosens up, about 5 minutes.

3. Add the chopped garlic, diced carrot (if using), and diced celery (if using) and cook for an additional 2-3 minutes, or until softened.

4. Stir in the frozen peas, dried thyme, dried rosemary, and smoked paprika (if using). Cook for an extra minute.

5. Flavor with salt and black pepper to taste.

6. Pour the leftover lentil soup into the skillet with the veggies and stir to combine.

7. Transfer the mixture to a baking dish suited for oven use.

8. Top the lentil soup mixture with the mashed potatoes, spreading them evenly to make a complete covering.

9. Bake for 20-25 minutes, or until the mashed potatoes are golden brown and bubbly.

10. Serve hot topped with chopped fresh parsley (optional).

Black Bean Burger Transformation: Black Bean Burrito Bowls (Serves 4):

Repurpose extra black bean burgers into delicious and customizable burrito bowls.

Ingredients:

2 tablespoons olive oil

1 medium onion, chopped 1 bell pepper (any color), diced

1 cup chopped veggies (e.g., corn, zucchini, mushrooms)

1 teaspoon chili spice

1/2 teaspoon cumin

1/4 teaspoon smoked paprika (optional)

Salt and black pepper to taste

2 cups cooked brown rice (or other grain of your choice)

2 extra black bean burgers, crumbled 1 (15 oz) can black beans, drained and rinsed (optional)

Chopped romaine lettuce or chopped cabbage (for the base)

Your favorite burrito bowl ingredients (e.g., salsa, guacamole, sour cream, shredded cheese, chopped fresh cilantro, sliced avocado)

Instructions:

1. Heat olive oil in a big skillet or pan over medium heat. Add the chopped onion and bell pepper and cook until softened, about 5 minutes.

2. Add the chopped veggies (corn, zucchini, mushrooms) and cook for an additional 3-4 minutes, or until tender-crisp.

3. Stir in the chili powder, cumin, and smoked paprika (if using). Season with salt and black pepper to taste.

4. In a different bowl, warm up the cooked brown rice.

5. Crumble the extra black bean burgers into bite-sized pieces.

6. To make the burrito bowls, start with a bed of chopped romaine lettuce or shredded cabbage in a bowl.

7. Top with the warmed brown rice, crumbled black bean burgers, cooked vegetable mixture, and any extra desired toppings (salsa, guacamole, sour cream, shredded cheese, chopped fresh cilantro, sliced avocado).

These leftover transformation recipes offer just a glimpse of the options. With a little creativity and these handy tips, you can turn your leftovers into exciting and delicious new meals, reducing food waste and saving you time and money in the kitchen. So next time you find yourself with extra food, don't toss it! Get artistic and discover the magic of leftover transformations!

PART 3: MEAL PREP MASTERY - BUDGET-FRIENDLY PLANT-BASED MEAL PREP

Welcome back to Meal Prep Mastery! This part focuses on the art of batch cooking specifically for plant-based meals, keeping your budget in mind. Batch cooking allows you to make multiple meals at once, saving you time and energy throughout the week. It's a great strategy for busy individuals who still want to enjoy delicious and nutritious plant-based meals.

This part kicks off with the foundation of batch cooking

CHAPTER 9: BATCH COOKING BASICS

Embracing batch cooking is a game-changer for busy individuals who value healthy and delicious meals. This chapter dives into the important steps to get you started with batch cooking plant-based meals on a budget.

The Benefits of Batch Cooking:

1. Save Time: By cooking multiple meals at once, you greatly reduce the time spent in the kitchen throughout the week.

2. Save Money: Batch cooking allows for efficient use of ingredients, minimizing waste and helping you stretch your shopping budget.

3. Eat Healthier: Having pre-prepared meals easily available encourages healthy choices and reduces reliance on convenience foods.

4. Reduce Stress: Knowing you have healthy meals prepped takes the pressure off during busy weeks.

Planning Your Batch Cooking Sessions

Planning is key to good batch cooking. Here's how to get organized:

1. Choose Your Recipes: Select a few recipes that are batch-friendly and fit your nutritional needs. Consider meals with similar ingredients to improve efficiency. Check out the future chapters for some budget-friendly plant-based recipe inspiration!

2. Make a Shopping List: Plan your grocery list based on the picked recipes. Look for sales and buy in bulk (when possible) for staples like grains and legumes.

3. Schedule Your Cooking Session: Set aside a set time for batch cooking. Aim for 1-2 hours, based on the recipes and your experience.

Essential Tools for Batch Cooking Success:

Having the right tools makes batch cooking a snap. Consider these essentials:

1. Large Pots and Pans: Choose a range of sizes for boiling grains, simmering sauces, and sautéing vegetables.

2. Sharp Knives and Cutting Boards: Invest in good quality knives and a strong cutting board for efficient prep work.

3. Sheet Pans: These are great for roasting vegetables, tofu, or tempeh in large batches.

4. Food Storage Containers: Airtight containers are crucial for keeping your prepped meals in the refrigerator or freezer.

5. Labels: Label your containers with the ingredients and date to keep track of your prepped foods.

Reheating and Storing Batch-Cooked Meals

Proper storage and reheating are important for maintaining the quality and safety of your batch-cooked meals.

1. Storing: Allow cooked food to cool completely before storing. Transfer them to airtight containers and store in the refrigerator for 3-4 days or freeze for longer keeping (up to 3 months).

2. Reheating: Reheat meals slowly on the stovetop over low heat or in the microwave using short bursts with stirring in between. Avoid overheating, which can affect taste and texture.

Additional Batch Cooking Tips:

1. Double Up! While cooking, try doubling a recipe to have extra portions for lunch or another quick dinner.

2. Portion Control: When storing prepped meals, portion them out individually for easy grab-and-go ease.

3. Get Creative with Leftovers: Get inspired by Chapter 8: Leftover Transformations for turning leftovers into new and exciting meals.

4. Clean Up as You Go: Washing dishes as you cook reduces the post-cooking cleanup.

Embrace the Batch Cooking Lifestyle!

Batch cooking is a useful skill for anyone who wants to save time and money while eating healthy.

With a little planning and the tips provided in this chapter, you can create a batch cooking routine that fits your lifestyle and budget. Get ready to enjoy delicious, plant-based meals all week long with minimal work!

The next chapters in this part will provide you with a variety of budget-friendly plant-based recipes especially designed for batch cooking success. So grab your grocery list, plan your cooking session, and get ready to open the world of delicious and convenient plant-based meal prep!

CHAPTER 10: STAPLE STARS: BUILDING A BUDGET-FRIENDLY VEGAN PANTRY

Embracing a plant-based living doesn't have to break the bank! This chapter focuses on building a well-stocked vegan pantry filled with budget-friendly staples that form the basis of countless delicious meals. With these important ingredients on hand, you can whip up quick and healthy meals throughout the week without needing a trip to the store every day.

The Benefits of a Stocked Vegan Pantry:

1. Save Time: Having key ingredients easily available eliminates frequent grocery runs, saving you valuable time.
2. Save Money: Purchasing staples in bulk (when possible) and planning meals around what you have on hand reduces impulse buys and food waste.

3. Boost Creativity: A well-stocked pantry encourages culinary exploration, allowing you to create new and exciting dishes with easily available ingredients.
4. Peace of Mind: Knowing you have a base of items on hand provides peace of mind, especially on busy days when whipping up a meal from scratch seems daunting.

Building a Budget-Friendly Vegan Pantry:

Here's a guide to building your plant-based pantry without going overboard:

1. Start with the Basics: Focus on versatile staples you can use in a variety of meals.
2. Consider Your Needs: Choose ingredients that fit your dietary tastes and cooking style.
3. Shop Smart: Look for sales, buy in bulk (when practical) for frequently used items, and utilize store names for staples.
4. Prioritize Shelf-Stable and Long-Lasting Ingredients: Build a foundation of things with long shelf life to minimize spoilage.

Stocking Up on Grains and Legumes:

Grains and legumes are the workhorses of a vegan pantry, providing important carbohydrates, protein, and fiber. Here are some key players:

Grains:

1. Brown Rice: A whole grain powerhouse giving sustained energy. It's perfect for soups, stir-fries, and pilafs.
2. Quinoa: A complete protein grain with a slightly nutty taste. Enjoy it in salads, bowls, or cooked like rice.
3. Oats: A budget-friendly breakfast favorite, oats are also great for baking or overnight oats.
4. Pasta (whole wheat preferred): A versatile and satisfying choice for quick meals.
5. Couscous or Bulgur Wheat: These quick-cooking choices are great for salads, bowls, or stuffing vegetables.

Tips: Purchase brown rice in larger bags, and opt for whole wheat types of pasta whenever possible for added fiber.

Legumes:

Dried Beans (e.g., black beans, kidney beans, chickpeas, lentils): Incredibly budget-friendly and versatile, dried beans offer endless recipe options. Soak and cook them at home, or utilize canned types for convenience.

Lentils: Packed with protein and fiber, lentils cook quickly and are great for soups, stews, and dals.

Tips: Buy dried beans in bulk and soak them at home for the most budget-friendly choice. Canned beans are a convenient option, but watch out for added sodium. Rinse canned beans before using to lower sodium content.

Essential Canned Goods and Frozen Staples:

Canned and frozen choices offer convenience and affordability, allowing you to add variety and nutrients to your meals:

Canned Goods:

Diced Tomatoes: A delicious base for countless sauces, soups, and stews. Opt for diced tomatoes with no extra salt.

Chickpeas (garbanzo beans): These flexible legumes can be enjoyed in salads, curries, dips like hummus, or roasted for a crunchy snack.

Black Beans: A protein and fiber powerhouse, black beans are great for tacos, burritos, soups, and salads.

Kidney Beans: These dark red beans add a distinctive taste to chili, stews, and vegetarian "meatloaf."

Coconut Milk: A creamy dairy-free option for curries, soups, and smoothies. Choose unsweetened versions.

Vegetable Broth: A delicious base for soups, stews, and sauces.

Tips: Look for canned goods with BPA-free wrapping and opt for low-sodium or no-salt-added options whenever possible.

Frozen Staples:

Frozen Vegetables: Affordable and readily available, frozen vegetables offer a variety of choices for quick and easy meals. Choose frozen veggies with no added sauce or salt.

Frozen Fruits: Stock up on frozen berries, mangoes, or pineapples for smoothies, smoothie bowls, or baking.

Frozen Edamame: A convenient source of protein and healthy fats, great for adding to salads, stir-fries, or bowls.

Tips: Look for frozen vegetables that are flash-frozen at their peak freshness to protect nutrients. Frozen veggies are a great way to add vitamins and antioxidants to your diet year-round.

Beyond the Basics: Plant-Based Pantry Boosters

Once you've created a foundation of staples, consider adding these extras to elevate your vegan pantry:

Plant-Based Milk (e.g., almond milk, soy milk): Perfect for smoothies, sauces, and adding creaminess to meals. Opt for unsweetened versions.

Nut Butters (peanut butter, almond butter): A source of healthy fats and protein, nut butters are great for sandwiches, snacks, or adding flavor to sauces. Choose natural types with minimal added ingredients.

Seeds (chia seeds, flaxseeds): These tiny powerhouses are packed with nutrients and add a textural element to recipes. Try adding them to oatmeal, smoothies, or yogurt replacements.

Dried Herbs and Spices: A small investment in spices can turn simple dishes into flavorful creations. Start with a basic set like oregano, basil, cumin, chili powder, and paprika, and expand your collection as you try new cuisines.

Healthy Fats (e.g., olive oil, avocado oil): Essential for adding taste and promoting satiety, healthy fats are crucial for a balanced vegan diet.

Tips: Purchase spices in whole form whenever possible for maximum flavor and grind them yourself for the best taste. Store spices in airtight packages in a cool, dark place to maintain their potency.

Maintaining Your Vegan Pantry:

Rotate Stock: Regularly check your pantry and use older things first to avoid spoilage.

Shop with a List: Planning your meals and making a grocery list helps you avoid impulse purchases and ensures you're buying what you need.

Embrace Versatility: When considering new purchases, think about how an ingredient can be used in various dishes to maximize its worth.

CHAPTER 11: PLANNING FOR SUCCESS: MASTERING PLANT-BASED MEAL PREP

The key to efficient plant-based meal prep lies in planning. This chapter equips you with valuable strategies for making a meal prep plan that fits your lifestyle and dietary needs while maximizing efficiency and budget.

Creating a Plant-Based Meal Prep Plan:

Planning your meals ahead of time sets you up for success with plant-based group cooking. Here's how to get started:

- **Consider Your Time Commitment:** Be realistic about how much time you can spend on batch cooking each week. Aim for 1-2 hours, based on the complexity of your chosen recipes.
- **Choose Your Recipes:** Select a few budget-friendly plant-based recipes that are perfect for batch cooking. Look for recipes with similar ingredients to improve efficiency. This chapter series will provide you with recipe inspiration in the following parts!

- **Make a Grocery List:** Plan your grocery list based on the picked recipes. Utilize the tips in Chapter 10: Staple Stars to build your shopping list around your current pantry staples.
- **Schedule Your Cooking Session:** Set aside a specific time for batch cooking in your weekly plan.
- **Account for Leftovers:** Consider how you might integrate leftovers into future meals to minimize waste (we'll explore this further in a separate part).

Utilizing Weekly Flyers and Sales:

Planning your meals around weekly food store flyers and sales allows you to stretch your budget further. Here are some tips:

- **Browse Weekly Flyers:** Check out flyers from your local grocery shops to see what's on sale. Look for deals on staples like grains, legumes, and veggies.
- **Plan Around Sales:** Choose recipes based on the items that are on sale that week. This is a great way to find new and budget-friendly plant-based options.
- **Stock Up on Staples:** If a staple ingredient you use frequently is on sale, consider getting a larger quantity to store for future use. Just be aware of expiration dates.

Leftover Integration into Meal Prep:

Leftovers are an excellent chance to get creative and minimize food waste. Here are some ways to add leftovers into your meal prep:

- **Repurpose Leftovers:** Get motivated by Chapter 8: Leftover Transformations! This chapter offers creative ways to turn leftover roasted vegetables, lentil soup, and black bean burgers into entirely new and delicious meals.
- **Portion Leftovers for Lunches:** When batch cooking, consider portioning out some of the cooked food for quick and easy lunches throughout the week.
- **Plan Leftover Integration:** While making your meal plan, consider how you might integrate potential leftovers from one recipe into another meal later in the week.

Creating Your Weekly Meal Prep Schedule:

Once you've chosen your recipes, made a grocery list, and planned around sales, it's time to build your weekly meal prep schedule. Here's a way to consider:

1. **Day 1 (or 2):** Dedicate this time to your big cooking session. Cook the meals you've picked for the week.
2. **Assembly Days:** Throughout the week, spend a few minutes each morning or evening to

assemble your meals based on the pre-cooked ingredients. This might involve chopping fresh veggies, preparing sauces, or portioning out cooked grains and proteins.
3. **Leftover Integration:** As the week continues, incorporate any leftovers from previous meals into your lunches or dinners.

Meal Prep Essentials:

- **Airtight Containers:** Invest in a range of sizes to store pre-cooked meals and chopped vegetables. Opt for glass or BPA-free plastic cases.
- **Labels:** Label your containers with the ingredients and date to keep track of your prepped foods.
- **Reusable Food Wraps:** These are a sustainable option to plastic wrap for storing cut vegetables, fruits, or cheese.

Benefits of a Plant-Based Meal Prep Plan:

Planning your plant-based meals in advance offers numerous benefits:

- **Saves Time:** Batch cooking eliminates the need for daily dinner prep, freeing up time throughout the week.
- **Saves Money:** Planning meals and utilizing sales helps you avoid spontaneous purchases and food waste.

- **Promotes Healthy Eating:** Having prepped, healthy meals easily available encourages healthy choices and reduces reliance on convenience foods.
- **Reduces Stress:** Knowing you have healthy and delicious meals planned takes the pressure off during busy weeks.

Embrace the Efficiency of Meal Prep!

Meal prepping isn't about rigid plans or complicated recipes. It's about planning and utilizing tactics to save time, money, and eat healthier. By incorporating the tips and strategies described in this chapter, you can establish a plant-based meal prep routine that fits your lifestyle and dietary needs

CHAPTER 12: FROZEN FAVORITES: UNLOCKING DELICIOUSNESS WITH CONVENIENCE

Frozen fruits and vegetables are a game-changer for busy individuals who value healthy and delicious meals. Often flash-frozen at peak freshness, frozen produce offers a convenient, budget-friendly, and nutrient-rich alternative to fresh choices.

This chapter explores the power of frozen favorites in plant-based meal prep, offering recipe inspiration and practical tips for incorporating them into your weekly routine.

The Power of Frozen Vegetables and Fruits:

Frozen veggies and fruits are packed with vitamins, minerals, and antioxidants. The flash-freezing process used by most manufacturers locks in essential nutrients, making frozen produce a great choice for keeping a balanced diet.

Benefits of Using Frozen Produce in Meal Prep:

- **Convenience:** Frozen fruits and veggies are pre-washed and chopped, saving you valuable prep time in the kitchen.
- **Affordability:** Frozen produce is usually more affordable than fresh options, especially when considering out-of-season choices.
- **Reduced Food Waste:** Frozen fruits and veggies have a longer shelf life, minimizing the risk of spoilage and food waste.
- **Year-Round Availability:** Enjoy your favorite fruits and veggies throughout the year, regardless of season.

Meal Prep Ideas with Frozen Vegetables and Grains:

Frozen produce opens doors to a world of delicious and convenient meal prep options. Here are some cooking ideas to get you started:

Breakfast:

- **Power Breakfast Smoothie Bowls:** Blend frozen fruits like berries or mango with plant-based milk, protein powder (optional), and a touch of nut butter. Top with your favorite granola, chopped nuts, and a drizzle of nut butter for a full and satisfying breakfast.

- **Overnight Oats with Frozen Fruit:** Combine rolled oats with plant-based milk, chia seeds, and a touch of maple syrup. Layer in your favorite frozen fruit (berries, cherries, or peaches) for a delicious and nutritious overnight breakfast choice.

Lunch:

- **Quinoa Veggie Bowls:** Cook a batch of quinoa and pair it with a range of roasted frozen vegetables like broccoli, cauliflower, and bell peppers. Top with a flavorful tahini dressing for a filling lunch bowl.
- **Lentil Soup with Frozen Greens:** Prepare a big pot of lentil soup and stir in chopped frozen spinach or kale towards the end of cooking for an extra boost of nutrients.

Dinner:

- **Stir-Fry Extravaganza:** Choose a protein base like tofu, tempeh, or beans. Sauté them with a range of frozen vegetables like stir-fry mix, peas, and carrots. Serve over brown rice or quinoa for a quick and flavorful evening meal.
- **Frozen Veggie Frittatas:** Whisk together a simple egg substitute mixture with chopped frozen veggies like broccoli, onions, and peppers. Pour into a baking dish and bake for a

delicious and protein-packed frittata that's great for meal prepping breakfast, lunch, or dinner.

Tips for Thawing and Cooking Frozen Produce:

Thawing Methods: Frozen produce can be cooked straight from frozen for most recipes like stir-fries or soups. However, if a recipe calls for thawed produce, some quick ways include:

- **Microwaving:** Place frozen veggies in a microwave-safe bowl with a splash of water. Microwave on high for a few minutes, stirring occasionally, until thawed.
- **Cold Water Bath:** Submerge frozen veggies in a bowl of cold water for 5-10 minutes, or until thawed.

Cooking Methods: Frozen veggies can be steamed, roasted, sautéed, or used in soups and stews. Steaming or microwaving helps preserve the most nutrients.

Additional Tips for Using Frozen Produce:

- **Read Labels:** Pay attention to added ingredients when picking frozen vegetables. Opt for types with no added salt or sauces.

- **Seasoning is Key:** Frozen vegetables may benefit from extra seasoning after cooking. Experiment with herbs, spices, and a squeeze of lemon juice to improve their flavor.
- **Get Creative!:** Don't be afraid to experiment with different combinations of frozen fruits and veggies in your recipes.

Embrace the Versatility of Frozen Produce:

By incorporating frozen fruits and veggies into your plant-based meal prep routine, you unlock a world of convenience, affordability, and delicious possibilities. With a little planning and imagination, you can enjoy healthy and flavorful meals throughout the week without sacrificing precious time or exceeding your budget. So, stock up on your favorite frozen fruits and veggies, and get ready to explore the culinary potential of these freezer aisle heroes!

PART 4: COMFORT FOOD CLASSICS - VEGAN COMFORT FOOD ON A BUDGET

Welcome back to Meal Prep Mastery! This part focuses on remaking classic comfort food favorites in a delicious and budget-friendly vegan way. We all deserve a warm and satisfying meal sometimes, and this section shows that plant-based eating doesn't have to mean sacrificing taste or tradition.

Let's kick things off with Chapter 13, where we dive into the world of everyone's favorite childhood comfort food: mac and cheese!

CHAPTER 13: MAC AND CHEESE MAGIC (VEGAN STYLE)

Mac and cheese – a creamy, cheesy treat that brings back warm memories for many. But getting that same level of comfort and flavor without dairy can seem daunting. Fear not, plant-based friends! This chapter offers three delicious vegan mac and cheese recipes that are sure to fill your cravings without breaking the bank.

The Magic of Vegan Cheese Sauces:

The key to a good vegan mac and cheese lies in the creamy and flavorful cheese sauce. There are several methods you can take, each with its own advantages:

Cashew-Based Sauce: Soaked cashews blended with nutritional yeast, spices, and a touch of lemon juice make a surprisingly creamy and cheesy sauce.

Starchy Vegetable Sauce: Roasted or boiled potatoes, cauliflower, or sweet potatoes blended with nutritional yeast and spices make a naturally thick and flavorful sauce.

Nutritional Yeast: This deactivated yeast has a cheesy and slightly nutty taste, and it's a staple ingredient in many vegan cheese sauce recipes.

Classic Vegan Mac and Cheese (Serves 4):

This recipe is a great foundation for trying different flavor variations.

Ingredients:

12 oz (340g) elbow macaroni or other favorite pasta
1 cup (240ml) raw cashews, soaked for at least 2 hours (or overnight)
2 cups (480ml) vegetable broth 1/2 cup (120ml) nutritional yeast
2 cloves garlic, minced
1 tablespoon lemon juice
1/2 teaspoon Dijon mustard (optional)
1/2 teaspoon smoked pepper
Salt and black pepper to taste
1 tablespoon olive oil

Instructions:

1. Cook the pasta according to package directions. Drain and set away.
2. While the pasta cooks, drain the soaked nuts and rinse thoroughly.
In a blender, combine cashews, veggie broth, nutritional yeast, garlic, lemon juice, Dijon mustard (if using), smoked paprika, salt, and pepper. Blend until smooth and creamy.
3. Heat olive oil in a large pot over medium heat. Add the cashew sauce and bring to a simmer, stirring constantly.
4. Reduce heat and boil for 5 minutes, allowing the sauce to thicken slightly.
5. Add the cooked pasta to the sauce and toss to coat equally.
Serve quickly and enjoy!

Tips:
For a richer taste, add a tablespoon of vegan butter to the sauce while simmering.
If the sauce is too thick, add a splash of extra vegetable broth to thin it out.
Feel free to add a sprinkle of your favorite chopped fresh herbs like chives or parsley for extra taste.

Spicy Vegan Mac and Cheese with Jalapeños (Serves 4):

Spice up your mac and cheese with this flavorful version!

Ingredients:
1. Follow the recipe for Classic Vegan Mac and Cheese above.
2. In addition to the mentioned ingredients, you will need:
- 1 small jalapeño pepper, seeded and finely chopped (adjust according to spice taste)
- 1/4 teaspoon chili spice

Instructions:

1. Follow steps 1-3 from the Classic Mac and Cheese recipe.
2. Add the chopped jalapeño pepper and chili powder to the mixer along with the other sauce ingredients.
3. Continue with steps 4-7 from the Classic Mac and Cheese recipe.

Tips:
1. If you prefer a milder form, remove the seeds from the jalapeño before chopping.
2. For an extra smoky taste, add a pinch of smoked paprika to the sauce.

Creamy Pumpkin Mac and Cheese (Seasonal - Serves 4):

This seasonal twist on mac and cheese is great for fall and winter comfort food cravings.

Ingredients:

• Follow the recipe for Classic Vegan Mac and Cheese above.
• In addition to the mentioned ingredients, you will need:
• 1 cup (240ml) cooked and mashed pumpkin puree
• 1/4 teaspoon ground nutmeg
• 1/4 teaspoon dried cinnamon

Instructions:

1. Follow steps 1-3 from the Classic Mac and Cheese
2. Add the cooked and mashed pumpkin puree, nutmeg, and cinnamon to the mixer along with the other sauce ingredients. Blend until smooth and creamy.
3. Continue with steps 4-7 from the Classic Mac and Cheese recipe.

Tips:
• To roast your own pumpkin puree, simply cut a small pumpkin in half, scoop out the seeds, and roast cut-side down in a preheated oven at 400°F (200°C) for about 45 minutes, or until soft. Once cool, scoop out the meat and blend until smooth.
• For a richer taste, add a tablespoon of vegan butter to the sauce while simmering.
• A sprinkle of toasted pumpkin seeds or chopped nuts adds a nice textural contrast to this creamy mac and cheese.

Beyond the Basics: Vegan Mac and Cheese Variations:

These ideas are just a starting point! Feel free to experiment with different ingredients and flavors to make your own personalized vegan mac and cheese masterpiece. Here are some ideas:

1. **Veggie Loaded:** Add your favorite roasted or steamed veggies like broccoli, peas, or chopped spinach to the cooked pasta before tossing with the cheese sauce.
2. **Herbacious Twist:** Stir in a handful of chopped fresh herbs like dill, chives, or parsley for a bright and flavorful version.
3. **Spicy and Smoky:** Add a chipotle pepper in adobo sauce (minced) to the mixer with the other sauce ingredients for a smoky and spicy kick.
4. **Nutritional Boost:** Throw in a cup of cooked lentils or chopped tempeh for an extra protein punch.

The Joy of Vegan Comfort Food:

These vegan mac and cheese recipes prove that plant-based eating doesn't have to be all about suffering. With a little imagination and these delicious recipes, you can enjoy all your favorite comfort food classics in a cruelty-free and budget-friendly way. So, grab your favorite pasta, fire up the machine, and get ready to indulge in a warm and satisfying vegan mac and cheese experience!

CHAPTER 14: SOUPS AND STEWS THAT SATISFY: PLANT-BASED COMFORT IN A BOWL

After a long day outside, there's nothing better than a hot bowl of soup or stew. This chapter goes over three rich and tasty vegan soup and stew recipes that will warm you up from the inside out. These recipes are also cheap and good for animals.

Why soups and stews are so good:

For plant-based meal prep, soups and stews are great choices. They're usually easy on the wallet, quick and simple to make in large quantities, and freeze well for later use. They're also very flexible, so you can add different kinds of veggies, beans, and grains to make a full and satisfying meal.

Making Vegan Broths That Taste Good:

Soups and stews taste great when they start with a tasty broth. Here are some ways to make a veggie broth that is rich and filling:

Vegetable broth. This is easy to find and makes a great base for most soups and stews. Look for low-sodium options whenever possible.

Homemade Vegetable Broth: For extra depth of flavor, try making your own vegetable broth by simmering vegetables like onions, carrots, celery, and herbs in water.

Bean Broth: The cooking liquid from canned beans can be used as a flavorful base for certain soups and stews, especially those having the same type of bean.

Minestrone Soup with Vegan Sausage (Serves 4-6):

This classic Italian vegetable soup is remade here with the addition of flavorful vegan sausage crumbles.

Ingredients:

- 1 tablespoon olive oil

- 1 onion, chopped
- 2 carrots, chopped
- 2 celery stalks, chopped
- 2 cloves garlic, minced
- 1 teaspoon dried oregano
- 1/2 teaspoon dried thyme
- 8 cups (2L) vegetable broth
- 1 (15 oz) can diced tomatoes, undrained
- 1 (15 oz) can kidney beans, drained and rinsed
- 1 (15 oz) can cannellini beans, drained and rinsed
- 1 cup (240ml) small pasta (like elbow macaroni or small shells)
- 1 package vegan sausage crumbles (optional)
- 1 cup (240ml) chopped fresh spinach or kale
- Salt and black pepper to taste
- Fresh chopped parsley, for garnish (optional)

Instructions:

1. Heat olive oil in a large pot or Dutch oven over medium heat. Add the onion, carrots, and celery. Sauté for 5-7 minutes, or until softened.
2. Add the garlic, oregano, and thyme. Cook for an additional minute, allowing the flavors to release.

3. Pour in the vegetable broth and diced tomatoes. Bring to a boil, then reduce heat and simmer for 15 minutes.
4. Add the kidney beans, cannellini beans, and pasta. Simmer for another 10-15 minutes, or until the pasta is cooked through.
5. If using, fry the vegan sausage crumbles according to package instructions and add them to the soup in the last few minutes of cooking.
6. Stir in the spinach or kale and cook until wilted.
7. Season with salt and black pepper to taste.
8. Serve hot, garnished with fresh chopped parsley (optional).

Tips:

- This soup is even more flavorful the next day, so consider making a large batch for meal prep.
- Feel free to add other vegetables of your choice, such as zucchini, peas, or chopped green beans.
- For a thicker soup, mash some of the cooked beans before adding them back to the pot.

Thai Coconut Curry Noodle Soup (Serves 4):

This fragrant and flavorful soup is packed with vegetables and rice noodles.

Ingredients:

- 1 tablespoon coconut oil
- 1 onion, chopped
- 2 cloves garlic, minced
- 1 tablespoon grated ginger
- 1 red bell pepper, chopped
- 1 green bell pepper, chopped
- 1 (13.5 oz) can coconut milk (light or full-fat)
- 4 cups (1L) vegetable broth
- 1 tablespoon red curry paste (adjust according to spice preference)
- 1 cup (240ml) vegetable stir-fry mix (or other chopped vegetables)
- 8 oz (225g) rice noodles
- 1 tablespoon soy sauce
- 1 tablespoon lime juice
- Fresh cilantro, chopped, for garnish (optional)

Instructions:

1. Heat coconut oil in a large pot or Dutch oven over medium heat. Add the onion, garlic, and ginger. Sauté for 3-4 minutes, or until softened.

2. Add the red and green bell peppers and cook for an additional 2-3 minutes, or until slightly softened.
3. Stir in the coconut milk, vegetable broth, and red curry paste. Bring to a simmer and cook for 10 minutes, allowing the flavors to meld.
4. Add the vegetable stir-fry mix (or other chosen vegetables) and simmer for another 5-7 minutes, or until the vegetables are tender-crisp.
5. While the vegetables simmer, cook the rice noodles according to package directions. Drain and rinse with cold water.
6. Add the soy sauce and lime juice to the pot and stir to combine.
7. To serve, divide the cooked noodles among bowls and ladle the hot soup over them. Garnish with fresh cilantro (optional).

Tips:

- This soup is easily customizable. Feel free to add your favorite protein source, such as tofu cubes, chickpeas, or tempeh.
- For a thicker soup, mash some of the cooked vegetables before adding them back to the pot.
- Leftovers can be stored in an airtight container in the refrigerator for up to 3 days.

Hearty Vegetable and Lentil Stew (Serves 4-6):
This protein-packed stew is a complete and satisfying meal in a bowl.

Ingredients:

- 1 tablespoon olive oil
- 1 onion, chopped
- 2 carrots, chopped
- 2 celery stalks, chopped
- 2 cloves garlic, minced
- 1 teaspoon dried thyme
- 1/2 teaspoon dried rosemary
- 8 cups (2L) vegetable broth
- 1 (14.5 oz) can diced tomatoes, undrained
- 1 cup (240ml) brown lentils, rinsed
- 1 cup (240ml) chopped potatoes
- 1 cup (240ml) frozen peas
- 1 cup (240ml) chopped kale or Swiss chard
- Salt and black pepper to taste

Instructions:

1. Heat olive oil in a large pot or Dutch oven over medium heat. Add the onion, carrots, and celery. Sauté for 5-7 minutes, or until softened.
2. Add the garlic, thyme, and rosemary. Cook for an additional minute, allowing the flavors to release.

3. Pour in the vegetable broth and diced tomatoes. Bring to a boil, then reduce heat and simmer for 15 minutes.
4. Stir in the lentils, potatoes, and frozen peas. Simmer for another 20-25 minutes, or until the lentils and potatoes are tender.
5. In the last 5 minutes of cooking, add the kale or Swiss chard and cook until wilted.
6. Season with salt and black pepper to taste.
7. Serve hot with crusty bread for a complete meal.

Tips:

- This stew freezes well, making it a great option for meal prep.
- Feel free to add other vegetables of your choice, such as green beans, corn, or mushrooms.
- For a thicker stew, mash some of the cooked potatoes before adding them back to the pot.

The Power of Plant-Based Soups and Stews:

These recipes showcase the versatility and comfort food appeal of plant-based soups and stews. They are budget-friendly, easy to prepare in large batches, and packed with flavor and essential nutrients. So, the next time you crave a warm and satisfying meal, consider whipping up a pot of one of these delicious vegan soups or stews!

Beyond the Bowl: Tips and Tricks for Soup and Stew Perfection

These recipes provide a delicious starting point for your plant-based soup and stew adventures. Here are some additional tips and tricks to elevate your creations:

- **Acidity is Key:** A splash of vinegar, lemon juice, or even a pinch of citric acid can brighten up the flavors in your soup or stew.
- **Fresh Herbs for the Finish:** A sprinkling of fresh herbs like parsley, cilantro, dill, or thyme adds a vibrant touch of aroma and flavor right before serving.
- **Spice it Up!:** Don't be afraid to experiment with different spices and herbs to create unique flavor profiles. Cumin, smoked paprika, curry powder, and chili flakes are all great options for adding depth and warmth.
- **Leftover Magic:** Soups and stews are perfect for reviving with leftovers. Toss in cooked grains like quinoa or brown rice, leftover roasted vegetables, or even shredded vegan meat alternatives for a completely new flavor experience.
- **Bread for Dipping:** Crusty bread or toasted baguette slices are the perfect

accompaniment for dipping into a hearty soup or stew.

Embrace the Versatility of Plant-Based Soups and Stews:

Plant-based soups and stews offer endless possibilities for exploration. With a little creativity and these recipes as inspiration, you can create a world of flavorful and satisfying meals that are kind to your body and budget. So grab your favorite vegetables, legumes, and spices, and get ready to discover the comfort and joy of plant-based soups and stews!

CHAPTER 15: VEGAN SHEPHERD'S PIE ON A BUDGET: A HEARTY CLASSIC REIMAGINED

Shepherd's pie, that soothing casserole of ground lamb nestled beneath a creamy mashed potato crust, holds a special place in many hearts. But for those living a plant-based lifestyle, the traditional recipe can feel off-limits. Fear not! This chapter shows a delicious and budget-friendly vegan shepherd's pie that captures the essence of the classic without the meat.

The Power of Plant-Based Shepherd's Pie:

Vegan shepherd's pie offers a fantastic alternative to the standard version. Here's why you'll love it:

Hearty and Satisfying: This dish is packed with protein-rich lentils and veggies, ensuring it keeps you feeling full and energized.

Budget-Friendly: Lentils are an affordable source of protein, making this a budget-conscious meal choice.

Flavorful and Versatile: The base recipe can be easily customized with different vegetables and spices, allowing for endless flavor exploration.

Perfect for Meal Prep: This dish reheats beautifully, making it ideal for meal prepping lunches or dinners throughout the week.

Building a Flavorful Vegan "Meat" Filling:

The key to a good vegan shepherd's pie lies in the savory and satisfying filling. Here are some tips for making a delicious base:

Lentils are the Stars: Brown lentils are a great choice for this recipe due to their texture and earthy taste. Ensure they are cooked until tender but keep a slight bite.

Embrace the Veggies: Don't be shy with the veggies! Chopped onions, carrots, celery, mushrooms, and peas are all standard additions. Feel free to try with other seasonal favorites like corn, green beans, or bell peppers.

Spice it Up!: Aromatic spices like thyme, rosemary, and smoked paprika add depth and warmth to the center. Consider a splash of soy sauce or tamari for a touch of umami flavor.

Creating a Creamy Vegan Mashed Potato Topping:

The creamy mashed potato topping is just as important as the spicy filling. Here are some tips for getting the perfect texture and flavor:

Starchy Potato Choices: Potatoes like russet or Yukon Gold are ideal choices for mashing as they provide a smooth and creamy feel.

Non-Dairy Milk Magic: Opt for unsweetened plant-based milk like almond milk, soy milk, or nut milk to achieve a creamy consistency without dairy.

Seasoning is Key: Don't underestimate the power of salt, pepper, and a touch of vegan butter or olive oil for a flavorful and filling mash.

Classic Vegan Shepherd's Pie (Serves 4-6):

This recipe offers a solid foundation for exploring your own vegan shepherd's pie variations.

Ingredients:

For the Filling:
1 tablespoon olive oil
1 onion, chopped 2 carrots, chopped 2 celery stalks, chopped 2 cloves garlic, minced 1 cup (240ml) brown lentils, rinsed 4 cups (1L) vegetable broth
1 (14.5 oz) can diced tomatoes, undrained
1 cup (240ml) frozen peas
1 tablespoon tomato sauce
1 teaspoon dried thyme
1/2 teaspoon dried rosemary
Salt and black pepper to taste

For the Mashed Potato Topping:

4 big potatoes (russet or Yukon Gold), peeled and cubed
1 cup (240ml) unsweetened plant-based milk
2 tablespoons vegan butter (or olive oil)
Salt and black pepper to taste

Instructions:

Prepare the Filling: Heat olive oil in a large pan or Dutch oven over medium heat. Add the onion, carrots, and celery. Sauté for 5-7 minutes, or until it loosens up.
Add the garlic and cook for an additional minute, allowing the spices to release.
Stir in the rinsed lentils, veggie broth, diced tomatoes, frozen peas, tomato paste, thyme, and rosemary. Bring to a boil, then reduce heat and simmer for 20-25 minutes, or until the lentils are soft but still hold their shape. Spice up with salt and pepper to taste.
Prepare the Mashed Potatoes: While the filling simmers, cook the cubed potatoes in a pot of boiling salted water until soft (approximately 15-20 minutes). Drain the potatoes and return them to the pot.

Using a potato masher or hand machine, mash the potatoes until smooth. Gradually add the plant-based milk and vegan butter (or olive oil) until desired smoothness is reached

Season the mashed potatoes heavily with salt and pepper.

Assemble the Pie: Preheat oven to 400°F (200°C). Transfer the lentil filling to a baking container. Spread the mashed potatoes evenly over the top, making a smooth and complete covering.

Bake for 20-25 minutes, or until the edges of the mashed potatoes are golden brown and the center is bubbly.

Let the pie cool slightly before serving.

Tips:

Leftovers can be saved in an airtight container in the refrigerator for up to 3 days. Reheat in the oven at 375°F (190°C) until warmed through.

For a crispy topping, broil the formed pie for the last few minutes of baking, keeping a close eye to avoid burning.

Feel free to add a sprinkle of your favorite vegan cheese alternative to the top of the mashed potatoes before baking for an extra cheesy taste.

Beyond the Basics: Vegan Shepherd's Pie Variations:

This recipe is a jumping-off place for endless flavor exploration! Here are some ideas for creating your vegan shepherd's pie:

Lentil Alternatives: While brown lentils are classic, try using green lentils or even a mix of different lentil types for a textural and flavor variation.

Veggie Extravaganza: Add in chopped mushrooms, zucchini, or bell peppers for extra vegetable goodness. Roasted veggies can also be used as a topping.

Spice it Up!: A pinch of cayenne pepper or a dash of chili flakes can add a touch of heat to the filling.

Flavorful Herbs: Freshly chopped herbs like parsley, chives, or dill can be added to the mashed potatoes for a lively pop of flavor.

Embrace the Budget-Friendly Versatility:

Vegan shepherd's pie is a great example of how delicious and satisfying plant-based meals can be budget-friendly. Lentils are an affordable source of protein, and the remaining ingredients are easily available and relatively inexpensive. With a little creativity and this basic recipe, you can make endless variations of this comforting classic, all while sticking to your budget. So, grab your best vegetables, spices, and lentils, and get ready to discover the delicious world of vegan shepherd's pie!

CHAPTER 16: EASY VEGAN CHILI DELIGHTS: A COMFORT FOOD CLASSIC GOES PLANT-BASED

There's something obviously comforting about a steaming bowl of chili on a chilly day. Packed with beans, veggies, and spices, it's a hearty and satisfying meal that warms you from the inside out. This chapter dives into three delicious and easy vegan chili recipes that are great for busy weeknights or cozy weekends.

The Magic of Vegan Chili:

Vegan chili offers a fantastic alternative to the traditional meat-based form. Here's why you'll love it:

Hearty and Satisfying: Packed with protein-rich beans and veggies, vegan chili keeps you feeling full and energized.

Incredibly Versatile: The base recipe can be easily customized with different beans, vegetables, and spices, allowing for endless flavor exploration.

Budget-Friendly: Beans are an affordable source of protein, making this a budget-conscious meal choice.

Perfect for Meal Prep: Chili cooks well in large batches and reheats nicely, making it ideal for meal prep throughout the week.

Building a Flavorful Vegan Chili Base:

The basis of a delicious vegan chili lies in a flavorful base. Here are some tips for making a rich and satisfying broth:

Vegetable Broth is Key: Choose a low-sodium vegetable soup for a healthy base. Consider homemade veggie broth for extra depth of flavor.

Spice it Up!: Aromatic spices like chili powder, cumin, smoked paprika, and oregano are necessary for a classic chili flavor profile.

Don't Forget the Acidity: A splash of vinegar, lime juice, or even a chopped tomato adds a touch of acidity that brightens up the tastes.

Choosing the Right Beans for your Vegan Chili:

Beans are the heart and soul of vegan chili, giving protein and texture. Here are some popular choices to consider:

Kidney Beans: These classic red beans offer a hearty texture and a slightly earthy taste.
Black Beans: They provide a smooth texture and a slightly sweet taste.
Pinto Beans: A good all-around bean choice, pinto beans have a slightly nutty taste and a creamy texture.
Cannellini Beans: These white beans add a creamy texture and a mild taste. Feel free to mix and match different bean varieties for extra variety.

Classic Vegan Chili with Kidney Beans (Serves 4-6):

This recipe is a great starting point for exploring different chili variations.

Ingredients:

1 tablespoon olive oil
1 onion, chopped
2 cloves garlic, minced
1 green bell pepper, chopped (optional)
1 (15 oz) can diced tomatoes, undrained
4 cups (1L) veggie broth
1 (15 oz) can kidney beans, drained and rinsed
1 (15 oz) can black beans, drained and washed

1 tablespoon chili spice
1 teaspoon crushed cumin
1/2 teaspoon smoked pepper
1/4 teaspoon dried oregano
Salt and black pepper to taste
Optional Toppings: Chopped fresh cilantro, vegan sour cream, chopped avocado, diced red onion

Instructions:

Heat olive oil in a big pot or Dutch oven over medium heat. Add the onion and green pepper (if using). Sauté for 5-7 minutes, or until softened.
Add the garlic and cook for an additional minute, allowing the spices to release.
Stir in the diced tomatoes, veggie broth, drained and rinsed beans, chili powder, cumin, smoked paprika, oregano, and salt and pepper. Bring to a boil, then reduce heat and simmer for 20-25 minutes, allowing the flavors to meld.
Taste and adjust spices as needed.
Serve hot in bowls with your favorite toppings.

Tips:

This chili is even more flavorful the next day, so consider making a big batch for meal prep.
Feel free to add other veggies of your choice, such as corn, carrots, or chopped mushrooms.
For a thicker stew, mash some of the cooked beans before adding them back to the pot.

Three-Bean Vegan Chili with Cornbread (Serves 4-6):

This recipe adds cornbread for a full and satisfying meal-in-one.

Ingredients:

For the Chili:
Follow the recipe for Classic Vegan Chili with Kidney Beans (above).
In addition to the mentioned ingredients, you will need:
1 (15 oz) can pinto beans, drained and rinsed
1 cup (240ml) frozen corn
For the Cornbread (Optional):
1 cup (125g) all-purpose flour
1/2 cup (75g) fine cornmeal
2 tablespoons sugar
1 teaspoon baking powder
1/2 teaspoon salt
1/2 cup (120ml) unsweetened plant-based milk
2 tablespoons vegan butter, melted
1 tablespoon olive oil

Instructions:

1. Prepare the Chili: Follow the steps for the Classic Vegan Chili with Kidney Beans, adding the pinto beans and frozen corn along with the other ingredients.

2. Prepare the Cornbread (Optional):
Preheat the oven to 400°F (200°C). Lightly grease a square baking dish (approximately 8x8 inches).
In a large bowl, mix together the flour, cornmeal, sugar, baking powder, and salt.
In a different bowl, whisk together the plant-based milk, melted vegan butter, and olive oil.
Pour the wet ingredients into the dry ingredients and stir until just mixed. Be careful not to overmix.
Pour the cornbread batter into the prepared baking dish.
Bake for 20-25 minutes, or until a toothpick put into the center comes out clean.

3. Assemble and Serve:
Serve the hot chili in bowls topped with a warm piece of cornbread (if using).
Enjoy with your favorite chili toppings, such as chopped fresh cilantro, vegan sour cream, chopped avocado, or diced red onion.

Tips:

- This combo is great for a complete meal. Leftovers can be stored in different containers in the refrigerator for up to 3 days.

- For a gluten-free version of the cornbread, use a gluten-free flour blend that is labeled as good for baking.
- You can also bake the cornbread separately in a loaf pan for a different appearance.

Slow Cooker Lentil Chili with Smoky Spices (Serves 4-6):

This recipe uses the slow cooker for a hands-off approach to a delicious chili.

Ingredients:

1 tablespoon olive oil
1 onion, chopped
2 cloves garlic, minced
1 green bell pepper, chopped (optional)
1 (28 oz) can crushed tomatoes, undrained
3 cups (750ml) veggie broth
1 cup (240ml) brown lentils, cleaned
1 (15 oz) can black beans, drained and rinsed
1 (15 oz) can kidney beans, washed and rinsed
2 tablespoons chili spice
1 teaspoon smoked pepper
1 teaspoon crushed cumin
1/2 teaspoon chipotle powder (optional, for a spicy kick)
Salt and black pepper to taste

Optional Toppings: Chopped fresh cilantro, vegan sour cream, chopped avocado, diced red onion

Instructions:

1. Heat olive oil in a big skillet over medium heat. Add the onion and green pepper (if using). Sauté for 5-7 minutes, or until softened.
2. Add the garlic and cook for an additional minute, allowing the spices to release.
3. Transfer the sautéed vegetables to your slow cooker.
4. Add the crushed tomatoes, veggie broth, rinsed lentils, drained and rinsed beans, chili powder, smoked paprika, cumin, chipotle powder (if using), and salt and pepper.
5. Stir to mix all ingredients.
6. Cover the slow cooker and cook on low for 6-8 hours, or until the lentils are soft and the chili has thickened.
7. Serve hot in bowls with your favorite toppings.

Tips:

- This chili is even more delicious the longer it simmers, so feel free to cook on low for up to 10 hours.
- You can easily customize this recipe by adding other vegetables, such as corn, carrots, or chopped mushrooms, straight to the slow cooker.

- For a thicker stew, mash some of the cooked lentils before serving.

Embrace the Versatility of Vegan Chili:

These recipes showcase the taste and ease of vegan chilis. With a little creativity and these recipes as motivation, you can create a world of flavorful and satisfying meals. So, the next time you crave a cozy and comfortable bowl of chili, don't hesitate to give the plant-based version a try! Your taste buds will thank you!

CONCLUSION:

THE JOYS OF BUDGET-FRIENDLY PLANT-BASED EATING

This book has studied the delicious and rewarding world of plant-based eating on a budget. We've delved into hearty soups and stews, a comforting shepherd's pie, and satisfying chili variations, all showcasing the versatility and flavor possibilities of plant-based cooking.

The Benefits of Embracing Plant-Based Meals:

Here's a quick recap of why plant-based eating can be a great choice:

1. Budget-Friendly: Plant-based proteins like lentils, beans, and tofu are usually more affordable than meat.

2. Packed with Nutrients: Vegetables, fruits, legumes, and whole grains are excellent sources of important vitamins, minerals, and fiber.

3. Versatile and Flavorful: Plant-based cuisine offers endless possibilities for exploration with countless flavor profiles and culinary traditions to find.

4. Sustainable Choice: Reducing reliance on animal agriculture can help to a more sustainable food system.

Final Tips for Budget-Friendly Plant-Based Success:

1. Plan Your Meals: Spend some time planning your meals for the week and make a grocery list to help you stick to your budget and avoid impulse purchases.

2. Embrace Seasonal Produce: Seasonal fruits and vegetables are usually more affordable and at their peak flavor.

3. Shop Smart: Utilize grocery store sales and coupons to stretch your grocery budget further. Consider getting dried beans and lentils in bulk for even greater savings.

4. Get Creative with Leftovers: Get creative with leftovers! Leftover veggies can be repurposed into soups, stews, or stir-fries. Leftover cooked grains can be used in salads or breakfast bowls.

5. Explore Plant-Based Staples: Stocking your pantry with staples like beans, lentils, rice, pasta, canned tomatoes, and different spices allows you to whip up a variety of delicious meals without needing a lot of additional ingredients.

6. Don't Be Afraid to Experiment: Have fun discovering different flavors and cuisines! There's a world of plant-based recipes waiting to be found.

Resources for Your Plant-Based Journey:

Here are some tools to help you continue your plant-based journey:

1. Cookbooks and Websites: There are endless cookbooks and websites dedicated to plant-based recipes. Explore cookbooks by budget-conscious cooks or blogs focused on affordable vegan meals.

2. Blogs and Online Communities: Connect with other plant-based eaters through blogs and online communities. This can be a great source of motivation, recipe ideas, and support.

3. films and Podcasts: Consider watching films or listening to podcasts that explore the benefits and joys of plant-based eating.

Embrace the Journey!
Remember, transitioning to a plant-based living doesn't have to be all or nothing. Start by adding more plant-based meals into your diet, and gradually increase them over time. The most important thing is to enjoy the delicious and satisfying world of plant-based eating!

ACKNOWLEDGEMENTS: A HEARTFELT THANK YOU

Writing this book has been a journey of exploration, discovery, and immense personal satisfaction. Before you dive into the world of delicious and budget-friendly plant-based meals, I wanted to take a moment and express my sincere gratitude to those who have helped make this book a reality.

Family and Friends:

My deepest appreciation goes to my incredible family and friends. Their unwavering support throughout this process has been invaluable. Their willingness to taste-test countless variations of soups, stews, and chili recipes (some more successful than others!) provided invaluable feedback and fueled my creative spirit. Their enthusiasm for my culinary adventures and belief in this project made all the difference. A special thank you to Tola Emmanuel

The Plant-Based Community:

This book wouldn't exist without the vibrant and inspiring plant-based community. Over the years, I've been deeply influenced by countless chefs, bloggers, and everyday individuals who have generously shared their knowledge, recipes, and passion for plant-based eating. Whether it was a groundbreaking cookbook, a beautifully photographed blog post, or a supportive comment on an online forum, these interactions fueled my enthusiasm and broadened my understanding of plant-based cuisine.

My journey began years ago when I was concerned about the limitations of a plant-based diet. Would it be flavorful? Could I still enjoy satisfying and hearty meals? However, as I delved deeper, I discovered a world of vibrant flavors, endless possibilities, and a renewed sense of well-being.

One of the most inspiring aspects of the plant-based community is the emphasis on creativity and resourcefulness. Learning how to create delicious meals from readily available and affordable ingredients was a revelation. This book aims to translate that very spirit – showcasing the accessibility and joy of plant-based eating for anyone, regardless of budget or culinary experience.

In Closing:

As you embark on your own plant-based culinary journey, remember, this is a chance to explore, experiment, and discover what works best for you. There's no one-size-fits-all approach. Embrace the process, have fun in the kitchen, and don't be afraid to get creative! With a little inspiration and these recipes as a starting point, I have no doubt you'll discover the immense joy and satisfaction that plant-based eating has to offer.

Thank you for joining me on this journey!

Warmly,
Maryann D. Lang